A Southern Girl's Guide to Plant-Based Eating

Recipes from the Vegan Soul that Won't Make You Broke!

CAMETRIA HILL

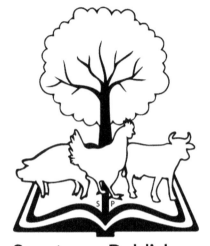

Sanctuary Publishers

Copyright © 2018 Sanctuary Publishers

ISBN-13: 978-0-9989946-2-8

Published by Sanctuary Publishers
www.sanctuarypublishers.com

-A Book Publisher That Gives Back-

Every book sold supports marginalized communities.

Cover Design & Illustrations: Danae Silva Montiel
Photography: Sarah Lockhart, Ryon:Lockhart Photography

This book is intended as general information only and should not replace professional medical or dietary advice. Although every effort has been taken to ensure that the information is accurate, each person's health and dietary needs are unique. Therefore, a qualified health care provider should always be consulted before any change in diet, physical activity, or other lifestyle change. This book is sold with the understanding that the author and publisher do not assume and hereby disclaim any liability to any party for any loss, damage, or disruption caused by errors or omissions, whether such errors or omissions result from negligence, accident, or any other cause.

DEDICATION

To my loving mother and number-one fan, Carrie Brooks (Sorry, Danny! Momma outranks you). Momma, you are the living embodiment of unconditional love.

I am what I am because of you.

To my grandma, Retta Hill, who made everything taste banging (I'm talking gourmet Kool-Aid, y'all). Thank you for teaching me how to put the soul in cooking.

I am grateful I inherited your cooking chops. I love you!

To the memory of my four-legged angel, Lex, who still makes me wanna be a better human every day.

CONTENTS

ACKNOWLEDGMENTS

I would like to thank all of the wonderful people without whose talents, support, and love, this book would not be possible.

Thank you to my publisher and birthday twin, Julia Feliz. Thank you for bringing my vision to life. You allowed me to stay true to my vision while stretching myself to make this book as accessible, concise, and informative as possible. You allowed me a vessel for spreading the food traditions I hold so dear and sharing them with people around the world. Thank you for your guidance and patience.

Thank you to my awesome and talented photographer, Sarah Lockhart— another birthday twin! You truly captured my food in a way that allowed each dish to shine. You brought out the best in me, as well, and I am humbled by your talent.

To my graphic designer, Danae Silva Montiel, thank you for creating a wonderfully eye-popping and attention-grabbing cover and the design sprinkles throughout the pages, which make this book that much more special.

To my fellow "Masterminds," Marino Benedetto and Nikki Daye. You were both with me from the very beginning, when I approached you with a dream that started with an ambitious idea to write an e-cookbook in 30 days. Thank you for motivating me and holding me accountable every step of the way. I love y'all!

Thank you to my partner and permanent recipe taste-tester, Kat Moore. Your love, support, and sacrifice are the only reasons this book could come to life. I love you!

Last but not least, to the stars of this book, my dear family: the Hill, Gorman, and Brooks families. Thank you for the traditions and memories that form part of my life's journey, which I now get to share with the rest of this world. Y'all continue to touch my life with memories and ground me.

I love you all!

PREFACE

ALLOW ME TO INTRODUCE MYSELF

I used to have a love-hate relationship with food. I always loved food but felt like it hated me. I was a big-boned kid, and, as my momma always said, "big thighs run in our family!" Bless her heart. Tired of going to stores and not finding my size, I decided I wanted to do something about it and take charge of my health. This helped me become fully vegetarian during my teenage years, despite having dabbled in it during my pre-teen years after witnessing some disturbing animal carcasses while on a school field trip to a ranch and butchering floor in Texas (by the way, that's where I'm from!). At that time, I was still growing in my convictions and ended up backtracking at an event at which I couldn't find vegetarian options.

Fast forward to a couple of years later. When I finally made the commitment and became a vegetarian, I wanted to fully immerse myself in it and make sure I was doing it right. I started to learn that there are illnesses directly linked to the food we eat (particularly animal-based foods) and when I looked around me with this new knowledge, I realized that many people in my own family were on medications for these types of diseases. I knew people on all sides of the family (even those only related to me through marriages) that were on medication for high blood pressure, cholesterol, and diabetes. Some of these people weren't much older than I am! While I am still curvy and love all of my curves, I finally understood that what you get out of your body is based on what you put into your body, and I did not want to end up with preventable diseases and on medication. At this point, I had learned that these diseases could possibly be reversed or improved through plant-based diets for some people, so I made a commitment to myself and never strayed from my vegetarianism.

About a decade later, my initial goal with veganism was to simply do a ninety-day "detox" and go back to my egg-loving ways afterwards. However, after watching a powerful video by a vegan activist on YouTube, which focused on the egg and dairy industries and the hidden cruelties that most of us don't get to see, once the credits rolled, I never looked back. I felt like a fog had been lifted. The video showed me the harsh realities of what I was unintentionally contributing to with my six-eggs-a-day habit. I didn't know that male chicks were viewed as useless, and thus ground up alive as feed, for example. It's one thing to think one is doing the moral thing by choosing to be vegetarian and not eating animals because of how they are treated and killed. However, once I knew about the atrocities also committed by industries that exploit animals for their bodily functions and byproducts, dared to look at the terror in the eyes of these animals and hear their shrills of fear and pain, I couldn't, in good conscience, go back to being a lacto-ovo vegetarian.

As I had done when going vegetarian, I researched veganism extensively to make sure I didn't accidentally consume something with animal byproducts in it. Apart from eating healthier and aligning my values with my actions, veganism kickstarted my interest in exploring new types of foods and recipes completely free from animal ingredients. This is when I began experimenting with recipes from my upbringing in Texas.

As a personal chef and restaurant consultant, I now get to fuse my love for my new lifestyle with the food culture I was raised with in the South. I am grateful to be able to spread those fond food memories with others that didn't get the luxury of grubbing in my grandmother's kitchen.

I hope this book impacts your life in all the beautiful ways being vegan has impacted mine. You have to start somewhere, and, regardless of whether you are new to plant-based eating or a seasoned vegan looking for some Southern food inspiration, I am glad you are here.

Love,

Cametria Hill

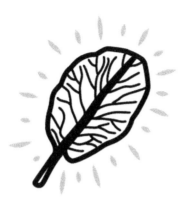

CHAPTER ONE

HOW THIS BOOK CAME TO BE

I grew up around food in the South. Evvvverrrrythang my grandma made was the bomb—everything! All of our events were centered around food. My stepdad barbecued every Sunday and my momma made a fish fry every Friday. Whenever we went to Big Momma's house on the weekends, we immediately went to the kitchen, where there were at least four different meals *even though she lived alone!* I have so many fond food memories that a certain scent from a dish can conjure a specific experience in my life.

When I became vegan, I knew I would be cooking only for myself, so my meals became another way to creatively express myself. I honed my cooking chops (outside of my grandma's culinary school) in several restaurants, pop-ups, commercial kitchens and food trucks in New York City. I was completely immersed in plant-based cuisine.

While working for a popular vegan food truck in Manhattan, I encountered someone who claimed, " Vegan food is rich, white folks' food!" as I explained to them about the types of vegan foods we sold and why. As time passed, the more vegan cookbooks and magazines that I encountered, the more I realized that, at that point in time, that person wasn't too far off the mark. Representation and diversity of multicultural communities were seriously lacking in vegan spaces, and plant-based resources seemed to focus on a specific type of cuisine.

In my quest for new resources that I could relate to, I stumbled upon the book *By Any Greens Necessary* by Tracye Lynn McQuirter MPH. As I was reading the intro from the book's sample on my Kindle (at the time, I only had the sample because I could not afford the whole book), one question that she asked really stuck out: "How many of you sisters know any older black women who are in good health?" That question was powerful to me because it took me back to the commitment I had made to myself when I first went vegetarian. I knew a lot of older black women in my life— grandmas, great grandma, aunts, aunties, and more— on medication. Sadly, I didn't know many over 45 who weren't on medication, and that's when it hit me: I had the tools, knowledge, and ability to provide healthier, plant-based alternatives to help my family and others regain their health. That's when *A Southern Girl's Guide to Plant-Based Eating* was born.

Whenever we have a family reunion and I make vegan food, although my family is heavy on the meat-eating, they go in and go hard; there's almost never enough! I always hear this statement, usually from my sweet Aunt Frances: "I could go vegan if I got to eat this every day!" I love to cook for people, but since I live about 1500 miles from my nearest family member, truthfully, I can only cook for them once a year. Therefore, this book is a way for me to empower people to be able to do this for themselves. It couldn't make me any happier if people from all ethnicities, cultures, and walks of life embraced this book and created their own food memories from the stories and foods of my culture and upbringing.

What This Book Is

The following pages are filled with recipes made up of all kinds of produce, glimpses of my Southern upbringing, love, and soul. Although this is a cookbook that will attempt to guide you through Southern plant-based eating, this is not a diet book. It is a book that will help you learn that it IS possible to change the way you eat to make your lifestyle healthier and more ethical, and will help you to see how. You don't have to compromise on flavor or taste!

I have attempted to use ingredients that you can easily find in grocery stores, so you don't have to worry about finding obscure and unaffordable ingredients for your meals.

You will find my "root-to-leaf philosophy" prevalent throughout this book, as it is inspired by the very premise of *Soul Food*: using the scraps and undesired pieces of food that were left over for the "help." You will find that I try to utilize as much of the plant as possible, from the root to the leaf. You can read a little more about this process and find other tips for plant-based cooking in Chapter 4.

If you are new to plant-based eating, you will find a jumpstart guide that will lead you through a week of meals and then help you plan future meals starting on Chapter 7. If you are a seasoned vegan, feel free to jump right into the recipes in Chapters 8.

As a bonus, Chapters 9, 10, 11 and 12 will help you continue on your plant-based journey through tips on eating out, finding support, and even getting more active as you go about your day.

First things first: I'm now inviting you into my kitchen. Kick back and enjoy!

Here's to creating your own food memories. Bon appétit!

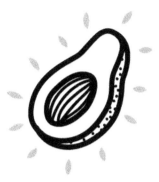

CHAPTER TWO

VEGAN 411, HUN!

You may have noticed that I have been referring to *plant-based eating* and *vegan lifestyle* as two separate things. That's because *plant-based* is in reference only to diet, while *veganism* is a lifestyle that forms part of the social justice movement complex. While this book focuses on plant-based eating, it is important to give you a brief overview of what vegan means, since plant-based eating is an intrinsic part of a vegan lifestyle. I chose this way of living for health and also to be inclusive of anti-oppression for all. The vegan lifestyle that I have been leading for over half a decade also helped inspire this book.

As an ethical lifestyle, veganism works to fight against nonhuman animal oppression from humans. It is a social justice movement with other animals as the reason behind it. That might sound odd if you are new to this concept, but nonhuman animal oppression and human oppressions are actually interlinked. So, while I am also against human oppression, working against nonhuman oppression was a natural progression for me. While human oppression is very different to the oppression of other animals, nonhuman animals have been traditionally used to "otherize" (make "less than" or marginalize based on differences) womxn, people of color, and other oppressed communities, as well as to justify their oppression. Therefore, when you stand up for animal rights, you are also working towards human rights. If you would like to learn more about these concepts, you can read more from authors such as Aph Ko and Syl Ko, Dr. A. Breeze Harper, Margaret Robinson, Saryta Rodríguez, Julia Feliz Brueck, and many others who have written about these connections on behalf of both humans and other animals.

As for the ethics of veganism, "If slaughterhouses had glass walls, everyone would be vegetarian." Although it is unclear who said this (Paul and Linda McCartney have been attributed with the quote, despite there being no record of it), I'm inclined to believe that this statement is true. I feel that most people are truly compassionate and have a moral compass that, if shown the true atrocities that our nonhuman friends are forced to endure, would make them think twice about using them as food or harming them in any other way.

I grew up in a typical meat-eating Southern household, and even after going vegetarian for well over a decade, I had no idea that, for example, in the egg industry, day-old male chickens were ground up at birth simply for the fact that they will never be able to produce eggs. Our relationship to other living beings is not a kind or just one, and further atrocities like what male chicks go through are standard, legal, and can be further found in the animal agriculture sector, companies that test on animals, the entertainment industry (horse and dog racing), the clothing industry (leather, fur), and among nonhuman animal breeders such as "puppy mills" (adopt, don't shop!), to name a few culprits.

With regards to animals exploited and killed for food in the US, many feel that, since the government regulates the food industry, these animals must be treated well. Sadly, this is not the case. Animal welfare laws do not apply to animal agriculture, and they don't apply to turkeys, chickens and some other species *at all!* This is most discerning because "poultry" accounts for 89% of land animal food deaths each year. They are also maimed in ways such as having their horribly sensitive beaks clipped and their nails clipped so as not to the damage the other "products" (their cellmates).

If this is your first time learning about these issues, it can be difficult to believe how any of this could be true and how any government could allow such injustices to be the standard, so let's further look at the two laws that *do* apply to animal agriculture in the US. The first is called the **"Twenty-Eight Hour Law."** This law states that animals transported across state lines by land for slaughter only have to be unloaded every twenty-eight hours for rest, food, and water. That's like driving from Texas to New York! I've done that trip twice as a roundtrip, and even with the luxuries of an air conditioner, reclining seats, snacks, and Prince CDs, it was almost unbearable. Now, imagine being crammed in a stuffy, sweltering trailer with excrement of other animals— or, even worse, the bodies of dead ones next to you. (Keep in mind that this law doesn't apply to birds classified as "poultry," who aren't protected at all.)

The second animal "welfare" law applying to animals used for agriculture is the **Humane Methods of Livestock Slaughter Act.** This law requires that "livestock," such as cows and lambs, be quickly rendered insensible to pain before being slaughtered. The common method used to "render them insensible" is a bolt gun positioned on the head, which causes the animal to convulse. Again, this does not apply to farmed birds, and it exempts certain forms of religious slaughter. However, how other animals are *treated* is not the point since *exploitation, oppression, and slaughter are still exploitation, oppression, and slaughter.* Just because a method is 'fast' doesn't mean it is painless, or that the animals' last living moments aren't any less terror-filled (a guillotine is also fast). At the end of the day, painless or not, animals have their lives taken from them when they would still prefer to live, as any of us would.

What's in a Label?

In the last few years, there have been trends to label meat and other animal products used for food with buzzwords like "natural," "free-range," or "cage-free." Many people feel that purchasing these often higher-priced items correlates to how these animals are treated, but just how true are these associations? Let's examine this a little further with each label and what each currently means.

Natural: When you see this label on a package of cutlets, it means there isn't something in it that you wouldn't normally expect in food. However, what does that even mean in itself?!

Free-Range: This label has no legal definition for use on eggs, dairy, beef, or pork. The label creates images of open fields and animals enjoying their short lives out in the sun; however, that is not accurate. Large sheds packed with thousands of hens still count as free-range.

Humanely-Raised: This label is also subjective and based on whatever imagery a consumer has in their mind about what this means. I will ask you this, though: Is it ever humane to take a life that does not want to be taken? What part of "humane" encompasses a bolt to the head, or being hung upside-down while having one's throat slit?

Hormone-Free: This label means nothing with regards to the treatment of nonhuman animals.

Cage-Free: Arguably the prom-queen of misleading labels. With regards to hens, cage-free means that they aren't raised in battery cages in which hens are packed in a single cage. (Battery farms are the standard for this industry.) However, birds used for meat are still raised in crowded sheds and aren't roaming pretty green pastures waiting for their time to "surrender" their lives.

Whatever label animal-based food is given isn't the point. Nonhuman animals are exploited and have their short lives taken from them without regard for the fact that that they, too, are living beings and have a right to their own lives, free from harm. I am at the point in my journey where I do not see nonhuman animals as things or products. They aren't here simply to clothe, entertain, or feed humans. Nonhuman animals are also part of this world, and part of what makes the Earth all around beautiful and unique. I learned this much from my beloved and now departed Dachshund, Lex. He taught me about my own humanity through his unconditional love. No matter how my day is going, his compassion is why I try to live each day like the saying on my favorite shirt: "Be the Person Your Dog Thinks You Are." I have to ask, what makes us humans love and protect one type of animal but not the other?

The Benefits

Apart from being an ethical lifestyle, being better for the health of the environment and being better for our own health are just two of several benefits that making the choice to give up animal foods, products, and other forms of animal exploitation afford us.

Here is a quick summary for each:

In addition to the cost of animals' lives, the overall consumption of animals is causing irreversible damage to the planet's resources. According to a study titled the *Estimation of the Water Requirements for Beef Production in the United States* by Beckett and Oltjen (University of California, Davis, 1994), it takes about 2,500 gallons of water to produce 1 pound of meat (varies slightly depending on the conditions use to raise the cows), whereas plant-based protein alternatives such as tofu require much, much less water. A soy burger, for example, only has 7% of the water footprint of the average beef burger in the world, according to a study in the Journal *Ecological Indicators* (Ercin, Aldaya, & Hoekstra 2011).

Consider that people around the world, including in the United States, don't even have clean drinking water, and we are wasting it on an industry that isn't a necessity for human survival. In addition, according to a report by the Food & Agriculture Organization of the United Nations titled *Livestock's Long Shadow* (2006), 18% of all human-induced greenhouse emissions are due to animal agriculture. That figure is greater than that of the whole transportation industry! According to a report from the Agribusiness Accountability Initiative titled *Environmental and Health Problems in Livestock Production*, to make matters worse, animal waste and byproducts (including feces) are often stored in lagoons and contaminate drinking water sources of surrounding communities.

Manure from the animal agriculture industry is also a contributor of air pollution. Alarmingly, spray applications of liquified manure to surrounding fields are sprayed in large quantities and give off dust particles that carry toxic gases and can penetrate the human lung.

Animal consumption is not just a problem on land; humans are negatively reshaping water ecosystems, as well. The non-profit organization Oceana warns that global overfishing and unsustainable practices have led to the near collapse of fishing populations and ocean ecosystems. The organization also estimates that about 40% of the global fisheries' catch is discarded in favor of commercially-valued fishes to satisfy speciesist preferences. Millions more of other types of animals, like whales and dolphins, die as "bycatch." All of those animals simply die in vain.

This discussion is not meant to make anyone feel guilty. These are real issues hindering our planet's health and our own survival. The problems extend beyond our own personal health and quality of life, since other habitats, species, and human beings— particularly those in less-developed areas of the world— suffer the greatest for our direct choices. If you consider that we are only temporary stewards of the Earth, what kind of planet do we want our children and future generations to inherit? Do we want to leave a planet that is unhealthy and bears the scars of exploitation, carelessness, and destruction because of our collective inactions? Or do we want our legacy to be a thriving, beautiful, and fertile planet for humans and all other living beings on land, freshwater, and sea?

Plants for Better Health

What is the one thing in your life that is so important to you that you are willing to actively save your own life for it? That's a powerful question, right? I start off with this thought because when changing your lifestyle (or attempting to make positive changes), at times it feels like you are fighting a losing battle. You may even find yourself asking, "Why the Hell am I doing this?" I know I have! As I previously mentioned, apart from ethics, my lifestyle was worth changing because I didn't want to be another black woman on medication and suffering from preventable diet-related illnesses. Although veganism and plant-based diets are not a cure-all from every single type of ailment or for every single individual, the Academy of Nutrition and Dietetics (2016) reports that vegan diets "may provide health benefits for the prevention and treatment of certain diseases." Their most recent report on vegan diets concluded that "…vegans are at reduced risk of certain health conditions, including ischemic heart disease, Type 2 diabetes, hypertension, certain types of cancer, and obesity. Low intake of saturated fat and high intakes of vegetables, fruits, whole grains, legumes, soy products, nuts, and seeds (all rich in fiber and phytochemicals) are characteristics of vegetarian and vegan diets that produce lower total and low-density lipoprotein cholesterol levels and better serum glucose control. These factors contribute to reduction of chronic disease."

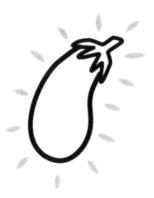

CHAPTER THREE

GETTING STARTED ON PLANT-BASED EATING

As I mentioned in the Introduction, what inspired me to write this book was my desire to bring awareness about the multitude of health benefits that eating a plant-based diet can provide. We all know that vegetables are good for you and have vitamins and minerals that we need, but just what *are* these nutrients and where can you get them? Here are some of the key vitamins and minerals that we need to maintain a healthy diet, and the foods they are found in:

- **B-complex**: Aid in energy release, growth, and metabolic functions; found in legumes, grains, etc. (B12 is found in some brands of nutritional yeast, fortified foods, and as a supplement.)

- **Vitamin C**: Helps the body absorb iron and may also boost the immune system; found in berries, citrus, leafy green vegetables.

- **Vitamin A**: Aids in bone growth, vision, cell division, and reproduction; found in dark-orange vegetables and leafy, green vegetables.

- **Vitamin D**: Aids in the formation of bones; found in certain fortified foods and through direct sunlight exposure.

- **Vitamin E**: Aids in neurological functions and as an antioxidant; found in seeds, nuts, avocado, and sweet potatoes.

- **Calcium**: Important for tooth and bone health, has a role in the clotting of blood and nerve impulses; found in broccoli and dark, leafy vegetables.

- **Magnesium**: Aids in bowel functions, muscle contractions, and nerve transmission; found in nuts, legumes, whole grains, and green vegetables.

- **Iodine**: Essential for the normal function of the thyroid and in metabolism regulation; found in certain table/cooking salts, seaweed, pulses and sea vegetables.

A Note about B12

Although B12 deficiency affects all people and is not a vegan-specific issue, people transitioning to a plant-based diet must pay special attention to getting the recommended daily amount (RDA) of Vitamin B12 required by human bodies– 2.4 micrograms (ug). It is important to note that a B12 deficiency can lead to anemia and nervous system damage. While it is true that animal derivatives are the largest source of B12, most vegans consume enough variety in their diets to avoid these health risks. This daily amount can be attained in a multitude of ways, which includes **fortified plant milks, some soy products, enriched breakfast cereals, and other fortified foods.** Examples of plant-based foods in the US that contain B12 include Living Harvest Hemp Milk, Coconut Dream Coconut Milk, Califia Farms Almond Milk, Marmite Yeast Extract Spread, Cashew Dream Milk, Bragg's Nutritional Yeast, and many more. Those outside of the US should also be able to access fortified plant milks and other sources of B12.

For those who do not consume fortified foods, B12 supplements are another suitable source for the vitamin. Unfortunately, plant foods that have been found to have B12 (such as nori seaweed and mushrooms) contain only trace amounts of vitamin B12 or only contain B12 analogues, which means they are not suitable sources for meeting our daily requirement.

Plant-Based Alternatives

Going plant-based these days does not mean going without; you will be amazed at the different types of alternatives available for meat, dairy, and even eggs! Here is a look through some of these alternatives to get you started. Types and availability will depend on your area, of course. Something to remember is that each brand is completely different, so if you don't like one, don't give up— you will find a new favorite in no time!

Plant Milks

- **Soy Milk** is perhaps the most similar in texture, taste, and uses as dairy milk, and is made from soybeans. This milk is arguably the best choice to use in coffee and perhaps the most readily available. As a small note, due to the many myths about soy out there, soymilk is perfectly safe and healthy to consume.

- **Almond Milk** is my preferred milk choice (I never liked cow's milk, even as a nonvegan, so this might account for my preference). It's lighter and great for smoothies.

- **Coconut Milk** is a thicker milk and mostly used in desserts, curries, and ice cream. I wouldn't recommend using this in coffee (unless it's a creamer) because it curdles in milk. There are brands of coconut milk (not canned) that are now closer to cow's milk, and some have suggested it is even closer to it than soy milk. You might find this to be true depending on the type of coconut milk you find in your area.

- **Other types** of alternatives include hemp milk, rice milk, oat milk, cashew milk, and pistachio milk. These may or may not be more difficult to find (if not available at your local grocery store, you will be able to find some in health food stores), but are helpful in case of allergy to any of the above. Just know that these tend to be pricier and not a close alternative to cow's milk.

Believe It's Not Butter!

The number-one ingredient in all things Southern, hands down, is a knob of butter. From bread to grits and green beans to butter beans, we subscribe to the notion that butter just makes everything better. While butter definitely adds a silky creaminess and a distinct savory touch in many Southern dishes, you can still achieve that in plant-based cooking with several easy-to-find alternatives. The key is knowing what purpose or function the butter had in that dish; this will help you decide on the best choice for your specific purpose. Here's a list of some common non-butter alternatives to use in your cooking, and their best applications:

Cooking Sprays: Most likely the lowest-calorie substitute for butter, these sprays are great to use as a butter alternative to prevent something from sticking to a pan (such as in baking). Just ensure that if are using a spray that says "butter-flavored," it doesn't have *whey* or *lactose*. The regular vegetable oil or canola oil sprays are fine.

Vegetable Oil: Plain good old vegetable oil (think canola oil) is definitely the most inexpensive and readily-available butter alternative, which will work really well in most baking that requires butter. The ratio is about 1 cup of vegetable oil per every 3/4 cups of butter that you would typically use.

Olive Oil: This is my favorite non-dairy butter substitute because it is so dang versatile! Olive oil helps me get a lot more bang for my buck! I primarily use this type of oil in place of butter when sautéing green vegetables, like green beans or kale.

Coconut Oil: Coconut oil has definitely been popularized in recent years, making it much easier to find and a lot less expensive than it used to be. This butter alternative is good for use in baking (it may add a bit of coconut flavoring to your food, so keep that in mind). I've used it in biscuits and didn't mind the slight coconut undertones.

Margarine: Although some margarines do have a blend of animal products in the oils, you can easily find some that do not. For the light margarines, for example, you can find brands that don't contain animal derivatives such as whey and lactose. Again, just double-check the label to make sure.

Plant-Based Butters, Spreads, and Cultured Butter-Style Blocks: There are several brands of vegan "butters" now found in most major supermarkets, in the refrigerated dairy section.

Egg Substitutions

My biggest hurdle to becoming 100% plant-based was my love of eggs. When you eat three kinds of eggs in the same meal daily, "love" may even be an understatement! You can imagine how important finding egg alternatives were to my transition, and I know I am not alone in finding it challenging to work around the use of eggs in cooking. Fortunately, there are several different foods that I and others have experimented with and conquered to get some pretty darned eggy results in vegan cooking!

Tofu is my go-to vegan substitute when it comes to recipes that need eggs for the sake of being eggs: recipes like scrambled eggs, egg salad, or an egg patty for use in a breakfast sandwich. Once you get the flavor blend down (check out the flavors in my **Eggy Marinade** on page 49), simply add a dash of turmeric for color, and you'll hardly miss eggs!

Cornstarch/Arrowroot are both readily available in the baking section of most grocery stores and work interchangeably. The combination of equal parts cornstarch/arrowroot and water works really well for binding in recipes, as they form a kind of slurry when combined. The typical ratio for one egg is two tablespoons of arrowroot/cornstarch, whisked with two tablespoons of warm water.

Ground Flaxseed whisked with water is affectionately known as "FLEGG." This is the go-to egg-substitute for use in vegan baking. To make one FLEGG, whisk 1 tablespoon of ground flaxseed with 3 tablespoons of warm water until the mix takes on a gluey texture. Let it set for 5-8 minutes before using in a recipe.

Chickpea Flour is becoming increasingly popular as an inexpensive, soy-free alternative to eggs. There are countless recipes that replace eggs with chickpea flour to make faux omelets and quiches.

Aquafaba/Chickpea Water is perhaps my favorite plant-based egg alternative. As you know, my food philosophy is "root to leaf" because I try to use every part of the vegetable to avoid wasting food. Aquafaba uses this same concept, as it is the brine (or water) that is left over from cooking beans/legumes. So, essentially, it's the chickpea water that's left over from draining the can. You use the leftover liquid instead of wasting it! Aquafaba can be used as a replacement for egg whites (it really works!). Some of the recipes in which you might use aquafaba include meringues, marshmallows, mayo, or egg-based cocktails.

But, Where Do You Get Your Protein?

The number-one question that all vegans get is, "How do you get your protein if you don't eat meat?" As if there is an epidemic of vegans dropping dead from lacking protein in their diets and eating animal flesh is the only way to stop it! Y'all, there are thousands and thousands of vegans living across the world and doing just fine. There are also plenty of huge-ass animals living quite happily on only plants. I'll get to the animal aspect in a second— hold my spot!

Now, I'm not sure where the idea that you can't possibly get protein if you don't eat meat came from, or that human beings require massive amounts of protein, but I do have my suspicions (Bacon, Bacon, Bacon, Bacon…ads everywhere!). In its report on vegan diets, the Academy of Nutrition and Dietetics (2016) confirms that, "Vegetarian, including vegan, diets typically meet or exceed recommended protein intakes…" So, where do vegans get their protein? Yup, plants.

Let's go back to Biology 101 for a sec (Getting flashbacks yet?). You *do* remember that humans are biologically classified as omnivores, right? This means that humans can thrive with or without eating meat. Humans are not carnivores by any stretch, or…When did you last find yourself chasing your food live, using your huge claws to catch it, and then eating it raw? Most likely, never (I hope!).

Now, all those big, beefy animals that actual meathead carnivores use to get their protein from? Are you ready for it? They are, technically, solely herbivores or mostly plant-eaters themselves! Some of the strongest and largest animals on Earth, that do not make part of anyone's meal, are also plant-eaters:

Cows spend much of their day grazing. They ain't eating their family members to get those curvy figures.

The Gorilla is arguably the strongest animal in the jungle, and is another tree-hugger.

Elephants, in all their majestic grandiosity, are also herbivores.

Essentially, when you fill up on beef, you are filtering the protein from plants through an animal.

Here are some examples of plant-based sources that are heavy on the protein:

- Peas
- Beans
- Chickpeas
- Lentils
- Tempeh
- Tofu
- Broccoli
- Hemp Seeds
- Chia Seeds
- Seitan
- Artichoke
- Spinach
- …and many more.

So, the next time someone asks you where you get your protein, tell them "kiss my grass!" Or just let them know that plants can be protein packed, too.

Hidden Animal Derivatives

When I was first making the leap from vegetarian to vegan, I wanted to be 100% sure that I was doing it right, as I have a very all-or-nothing approach. In my search, I was bewildered to find just how many hidden animal ingredients there are in all different types of food. I'm not talking about the obvious ones like cheesy this or bacon that. There were animal ingredients in things like Chex-Mix! It still astonishes me when something has milk or eggs in it, and it's not needed. To help make this easier for you, here are some ingredients that are or may contain animal byproducts:

- casein (dairy product)

- whey (dairy product)

- gelatin (from boiling the ligaments, bones, and skin of animals)

- red #40 (literal beetle juice made from crushed beetles!)

- natural flavoring (may be plant based but is often an animal derrived)

- albumin (comes from egg whites)

- pepsin (a digestive enzyme sourced from animals)

- tallow (fat of sheep tissue)

- isinglass (used in the production of some wines)

- anchovies (found in Worcestershire sauce and Caesar dressing)

- lutein (from egg yolks)

- stearic acid (found in some baked goods)

- glycerides (not always animal-based)

- oleic acid (not always animal-based)

- lactic acid (not always animal-based)

- suet (fat found in animal kidneys)

Tip: This isn't an absolute, but when you are reading a label, and it has cholesterol in it, it is likely that the item contains animal ingredients, since the only real source of cholesterol is animal products.

This list is a short overview of the types of ingredients and additives to look out for. Although there are others, if you try to avoid processed foods, you won't have to worry much about these types of byproducts. Either way, we have all been there, and label checking tends to become second nature after a few trips to the grocery store.

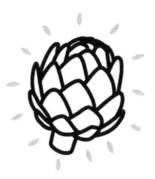

CHAPTER FOUR

PLANT BASED COOKING 101

A common misconception about eating a plant-based diet is that you have to give up so much and focus on eating salads all day long. This could not be further from the truth! Although folks often tend to focus on all the things that we choose *not* to eat, in reality, everything that you enjoy as a meat-eater, you can eat on a plant-based diet (Heyyyyyyy!). Being vegan and eating plant foods is not about depriving yourself. It's about really enjoying the flavors of plant foods without dousing them in animal fats. I'm not saying making some of those adjustments are second nature, but, as a girl from Texas, where all the vegetables have some type of pork matter in them, I'm here to tell you that you can still enjoy those same delicious tastes that you previously enjoyed.

What I have found on my journey through veganism and plant-based eating (and I use the word *journey* because every day I grow and learn more about myself in terms of compassion) is that there are so many possibilities to meals that I can create with the plant foods available to us. I have discovered so many fruits and plants that I would have never bothered trying or experimenting with, so my tastes have grown, and I am sure you will experience this as well.

In this chapter, we are going to look at flavors and general tips to tackle the recipes in this book. Think about all of the meat-derived meals you used to eat (I'm hopelessly optimistic and assume you have stopped or on your road to stopping!). No one goes over to a damn cow and takes a bite out of its leg! You know we season it with salt and pepper (plant ingredients), add some herbs (more plants!), maybe some aromatics like bell peppers and onions (again, plants!) and smoke the Hell out of it (a cooking technique you can easily duplicate in vegan cooking). When you really think about it, in meat cooking, it's all those plant-based ingredients that really make those flavors come alive. Once you get some of those flavor combinations down, why not use them to enhance the flavors of other plants?

Speaking of flava, here's a quick list of common flavor profiles and what they are reminiscent of:

Flavabombs Chart

This chart shows what spices and flavor profiles combine to replicate these non-vegan foods.

Chicken	Steak	Seafood	Pork	Eggs
Garlic powder	Cumin	Dulse flakes (sea vegetable)	Salt	Black salt / kala namak (find this online or at Indian markets)
Sage	Black pepper	Seaweed	Nutritional yeast	Bragg's liquid aminos
Salt	Sea salt	Old bay	Apple cider vinegar	Pepper
Thyme	Rosemary	Thyme	Peanut butter	Turmeric (bright yellow spice used in curries and mustards; found in the spice aisle)
Paprika	Rosemary	Cayenne	Liquid smoke	Garlic powder

Just so you know...

Bragg's Liquid Aminos is an alternative to soy sauce or tamari sauce used to season food and gives food a depth of flavor. It's also ok for a low-sodium diet. It comes in a bottle or spray pump, and a little goes a long way. You can find Bragg's Liquid Aminos in health food stores and in some grocery stores. However, if you can't find it or need a cheaper alternative, soy sauce is still fine to use instead (low sodium soy sauce exists, if you need that).

Nutritional Yeast (NOT baker's yeast) is a condiment that is yellow in color and comes in the form of powder or flakes. It is a very significant source of complex B vitamins. Sometimes referred to simply as "nooch," it gives different foods, such as vegan cheese, a tangy, funky, cheese taste. It is not a required condiment, but it will definitely bring your plant-based meals to another level. Most brands in the US have B12 in them, but check to make sure. You can find nutritional yeast in some grocery stores and in health food stores, but it is often cheaper if you get it online.

Flavoring Tips

Meats, cheeses, and animal-based sauces are sometimes used as the crucial part of a recipe used to give dishes their flavors. You might wonder how you can possibly make food that isn't bland and tastes good without them. Well, if you get nothing else from this book, I want you to truly get how to develop flavors and dispel that myth.

The following ingredients, used in many of the recipes in this book, are integral to getting flavors to POP!

Spices: Perhaps the most valuable of the products we put on food to please our taste buds are spices. In fact, spices are so valuable that they have served as currency at times, securing trade deals and even starting wars. Things like salt, regardless of whether in a savory or sweet recipe, release the intricate flavor of any ingredient or meal, so you will definitely find them in every dish in this book. (Sorry, I ain't sorry— salt is Southern gold!).

Herbs: My favorite things to cook with are herbs. They bring a certain freshness to any dish, and can give a dish a distinct feel. Think about cilantro; it is one of the backbones of great Mexican cooking. Fresh herbs give a certain aesthetic sophistication (as a garnish), but they can also define a dish. For example, if a dish is topped with basil, then you know you are about to enjoy the intricate flavors of Italian dishes.

If you do not have access to fresh herbs, you can use dried herbs instead. The typical ratio for fresh herbs to dry herbs is 3:1. Therefore, if a recipe calls for one tablespoon of a fresh herb, you can replace it with one teaspoon of the dried version (one tablespoon = three teaspoons). Dried herbs also tend to be less potent and fragrant as fresh, so if you aren't too keen on fresh cilantro (although I don't know how; I can eat that shit plain!), you can simply replace it with dried coriander.

Acids: Nothing brightens up a dish better than a little hit of acid. Whether it's a squeeze of lemon or lime or a splash of balsamic vinegar or white wine, acid is a great way to round out the flavors in a dish. Using acids is a trick you can use if a meal is feeling too heavy. For example, for a dish smothered in gravy, squeeze a little lemon into it to cut through the flavor. In addition, a little acidity will also help if a dish gets a bit too salty.

Heat: I love heat! Love, love, love it! I get that not everyone was eating jalapeño peppers when they were toddlers like me, but I feel a little bit of "picante" in a dish is an underutilized addition. When used properly, heat adds another depth of flavor to a dish. You can even awaken a good dessert with a pop of unexpected *capacin* (the compound that makes chili spicy!). Whether it's a sprinkle of cayenne or paprika in a fruit salsa or minced jalapeños added to a simple dish, adding heat to your plant-based dishes will bring even more complexity to your dishes.

Once you feel comfortable enough to experiment, when making the recipes in this book or cooking up your own creations inspired by what you learn from this book, try playing with the additions of the spices and herbs listed in the ingredients. Every individual will enjoy a specific amount of each, and once you find what that amount is, it will help to really make your food and flavors stand out. Get a good, solid balance of herbs, spices, acid, sweetness, heat, and oooh, mommmmy (that's my play on umami!)!

How to: Recipe Tips

My goal with this book was to make plant-based eating as easy, accessible, interesting and fun as possible for you. I wanted to use ingredients in my recipes that you wouldn't need help from the FBI to find. I definitely did not want to use ingredients that would require you to use your whole paycheck to buy them, either.

I also value your time. I strived to make the recipes the least labor-intensive as possible. In addition, I have gathered the following tips and insights that will make your time with this book even simpler. Whoop, here it is!

- **Read each recipe thoroughly before starting to cook it.** This will save you lots of time and energy trust me!

- **Whenever you are making a marinade, make extra and store it for later use!** This will give you a head start when making many of the recipes, especially if you are planning a week of meals ahead. Having extras will also give you a sauce to jazz up a pre-made plant-based protein you may buy from the store. To store the marinades, whisk together any extra marinade you may have and store it in a jar or airtight Tupperware-style container. A rubber spatula will help get the excess from the sides. Label the container with masking tape or label stickers with the date and store in the fridge. Try to use it up in 2-3 days.

- **Make your own aromatics blend!** Often times, you will find pre-chopped, diced *aromatics*, such as onions, garlic, bell peppers, or mirepoix (a blend of carrots, celery, and onion used to flavor stocks or soups) at supermarkets for a steep cost. The good news is that you can make your own blends from these to save time and money. To make your own, chop all of an ingredient when preparing a recipe and store the unused portion in an airtight container in the fridge. Alternatively, you can make little flavor cubes by placing the diced veg in an old ice tray for a pre-portioned measurement that you can use for soups or stews in the future.

- **On weekend days, if you have time, roast extra veggies and freeze them.** These will make easy side dishes during the week. They can also be used as the base for different grain-based bowls for weekday lunches. You can also make and freeze grains like rice to save time.

- **Save a little pinch of seasoning to add to the food directly before cooking.** For example, preseason the food laying on your cutting board before breading or sautéing. This will give even more flavor to your meal.

- **For safety, when you are cutting vegetables or fruit (especially big, sturdy ones), place a napkin or towel under your cutting board to prevent it from sliding around.** This is key in cutting things like large butternut squash or melons.

CHAPTER FIVE

SHOPPING, STORAGE, AND PREPPING

Shopping Tips

Whether you are new to the vegan game, just trynna switch it up a bit, or you just hate to grocery shop, it can be daunting or intimidating if you don't know what you're looking for. It's ok, though, 'cause I got your back!

Here are a few tips that will help you keep a little of that dough in your wallet and get the most bang for your buck:

- **Buy discount produce.** Grocery stores often wrap items in Saran wrap that will soon spoil and mark them down, so don't be afraid to scoop these items up! A really ripe tomato can make a damn good sauce and is sometimes better than waiting for one to ripen up.

- **Only get the amount that you need**! I know this sounds really obvious, but we are all susceptible to that "stomach bigger than the eye" phenomenon! It's better to start small than to buy too much and have it go to waste.

- **Stick to the list!** It is helpful to make a list of the items you need so you don't buy the wrong thing or something you don't need. Going to the store with a list not only saves you time, but monayyyy too! Can you say impulse buys? As they say, money is the motive, right? So, with all the extra money you don't spend on things you don't need, save up, and reward yourself with your choice of vice. Whether it's a mani, trip to the movies, or in my case, a guitar— keep ya damn money for you!

- **Buy whole foods!** As I mentioned before, processed foods are high-calorie with low nutrients, so, when possible, try to go with whole foods. Canned, bagged, frozen, or whole are all options available, depending on what your accessibility is. Dried (bagged) beans are cheaper than canned, but take longer to prepare. Frozen vegetables and fruit last longer, contain just as many nutrients and are sometimes cheaper than fresh ones. A large bag of rice is less costly than a single-sachet, microwaveable box of rice. So, if you can't access fresh foods all the time, there are alternatives that you most likely already buy that are just as good! The important thing is to try to avoid a diet full of overly-processed versions of food, such as ready-made meals, if you can do so, as these tend to be lower in nutrients yet higher in calories. However, we all do what we can with what we have!

Food Storage and Prep

I design my meals for the week based upon what will store the longest, what will go bad first, and how many ways I can multi-purpose a single ingredient. This is what I refer to as *strategic food storage*, which is helpful in saving money and cutting down on waste.

Depending on the fruit or vegetable, certain produce last longer and better when they are stored by themselves, in the fridge, or at room temp (and, in my case, on a hanging wire produce basket by my window!).

Here are some storage basics for various types of foods:

Green Vegetables: Vegetables such as broccoli and asparagus can be stored in the fridge for about a week.

Fresh Herbs: I usually store fresh herbs, such as basil, wrapped loosely in a damp paper towel and refrigerated in a plastic bag so they retain their moisture.

Root vegetables: Potatoes and yams store well inside paper bags in the pantry for about one to two weeks.

Lettuce & Greens: Whenever possible, I prefer to buy the whole heads or leaves of vegetables because they are typically fresher. You have more versatility with preparation with these than with the ones that are chopped ahead of time. If you do buy the ready-made packs, then go by the farthest use-by date, and use the leaves starting from the back.

Melons: You can stores these whole in the fridge for about five days.

Berries: They can be stored for about 3-5 days in the fridge. If available, you can purchase discounted berries and freeze them to use later for things like smoothies or jam.

Other Fruits: If you can, and unless this is your goal, store bananas and apples separate from other fruits, because they cause others to ripen faster!

Convenience and Meal Prep

To save money, I try to buy dried beans and grains. However, do note that they can be very time-consuming to make (unless you have a pressure cooker or a crock pot), so canned and frozen are perfectly fine to buy and use. The good thing about beans and grains, if you do make them from their dried versions, is that they store and freeze well, so you can make large batches. If I have extra time to spare, I'll usually make a few types of beans or grains and store them in the freezer so that they'll be readily available to make quick meals with throughout the week.

How to Freeze Beans and Grains

Beans:

- 1 pound of dried beans yields about 6 cups of cooked beans.

- Either soak the beans overnight in the fridge or *quick-soak* them (rinse beans, bring them to a boil in enough water to cover them, remove them from the heat, and let them soak for an hour).

- Cook them on medium-low heat for 60 to 90 minutes. Check on them and stir every 20 minutes. Then, add salt halfway through the cooking process (when they are slightly tender but still "al dente"). Note that if you add salt too soon, then they will get mushy!

- Once they are slightly tender and completely cooked, cool them completely. You want the beans to retain a bit of firmness since you will be eventually reheating them and want to prevent overcooking them.

- Portion them in a freezer safe bag with some of the cooking liquid, label, and freeze. You can save the excess broth for a stew or soup.

- When you are ready to use them remove them from the freezer and cook them on the stove-top.

Grains (Rice, Barley, Farro, etc.)

- They will store well for about 2 months.

- Cook the rice or grain according to the package directions (certain grains are quick-cook, so cooking times will vary) to the point of being cooked but firm ("al dente").

- Spread out the grain on a flat baking sheet to cool.

- Once cooled, portion, and place in a freezer safe bag. Seal the bags and roll out the extra air creating almost a vacuum seal.

- When ready to use, remove the grains and place them in the fridge or cook them right away. Do not fully defrost the grains because they will get "gummy." If you are making a stew or soup, then you can add the grains directly to the hot broth or liquid.

Other Tips

I always keep a large Tupperware container in my refrigerator for scraps. Things like onion ends, mushroom stems, and pepper tops make for a great base for vegetable stocks. They can also serve as inspiration for a great sauce or dip.

Whenever I'm making a recipe that needs half of a diced onion, for example, I go ahead and dice the whole thing and store it in an airtight container in the fridge for future use. You can even get an ice-cube tray and fill it with the chopped onion. This will give you a portioned-out base ready to use in a soup or stew.

If you have food scraps, such as shavings from carrots or the end of vegetables, you can use them to make a quick hearty salad in minutes. It's all about efficiency in the kitchen!

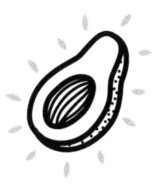

CHAPTER SIX

STAYING FULL AND SATISFYING YOUR CRAVINGS

In the beginning, when thinking about eating a diet that's heavy on the plants, it can be difficult to understand how one can get full on them. Trust me, I'm from the South, and I love, love, love to grub as much as the next girl (and didn't I mention I'm from Texas, where urrrrrrythang is bigger?). While transitioning to plant-based eating, I learned about a way of eating in which you eat more without it affecting your weight negatively. The premise involves eating lots of the right types of food, which, in other words, means getting the most bang for your buck!

The idea behind this concept is *volumetrics*: You bulk up your meals with lots of fruits and vegetables so that you can stay fuller longer. The idea is to load up with lots of foods that are non-starchy and nutrient-dense, rather than eating highly-caloric foods that are packed with empty calories. When referring to *empty calories*, I mean food that may contain a high number of calories, but very low nutritional value (think processed foods like chips, cookies, and all that goodness).

Examples of foods that you can add to meals that will help you to stay fuller for longer include spinach, broccoli, a handful of nuts, berries, apples, asparagus, sunflower seeds, and carrots.

If You Need a Fix: Tricks to Combat Those Cravings!

If you have ever been on a diet, you know the one thing that sabotages you the most is preparedness. The same principle applies when making the transition to plant-based eating or when adopting the vegan lifestyle. Being prepared will help you in situations where you are on the go, at a meeting, or simply at home and find yourself craving a bite. Although more and more vegan foods are becoming available, many convenient foods do contain some type of animal product. This is why it is important that you have a game plan, so you can help yourself truly succeed along with the reminder of your own personal "WHY?" for changing your lifestyle choices, including the way you eat.

Here are few things you can keep in stock to eat in a hungry pinch if you are on the go:

- a handful of almonds, cashews, or other nuts

- trail mix

- sunflower or pumpkin seeds

- hummus and pretzels

- fruit (fresh and dried)

- yogurt*

*Look out for plant-milk-based varieties, such as soy- or coconut-based yogurts.

These are just a few simple suggestions; however, as you continue to explore, you will find many more options depending on your tastes. I have also included a few snack recipes starting on page 95.

Comfort Food Swaps

When you're just getting used to the whole vegan thang, it's sometimes hard to know where to begin when trying to make a meal. Sometimes you just need access to your typical comfort foods. Luckily, many alternatives exist in major grocery stores.

If you can swing it, you can find vegan cream cheese, alternatives to block cheese, single slice cheese, vegan butter, and even plant-based meats and meals ready to cook or heat in a microwave.

Although it is nice to know these alternatives exist, you can easily recreate your own typical American go-to comfort meals. All you need to know is what to swap for the typically meat-centered part of the meal.

So, here you go:

American Meals Swap

Meat Version	Protein Swap	Add-Ons	Condiments	Other
Beef Tacos/ Fajita	Grilled Tofu, or Marinated Mushroom	Grilled Peppers, Onions	Guacamole, Hot Sauce, Pico de Gallo	Corn Tortillas & Cilantro
Cheeseburger w/ Mayo	Black Bean Patty or Portabella Cap	Lettuce, Red Onion, Tomato, Sprouts	Hummus, or Dijon Mustard	Toasted Bun, Large Romaine Leaf
Spaghetti w/ Ground Beef	Beef-less Crumbles, Mushrooms, Eggplant	Eggplant, Basil, Nooch	Pesto, Marinara	Pasta, Spiraled Veggies

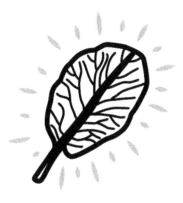

CHAPTER SEVEN

JUMPSTART EATING GUIDE & RECIPES

Now on to the reason you opened this book— the recipes!

I made it a goal to have interesting dishes that incorporated ingredients that can be easily found in major grocery stores. However, if for some reason there is a specific ingredient that you can't find, most of the recipes work well with a similar item. For example, if you can't find fresh basil, you can use dried basil instead (refer to Chapter 4 for a reminder of the fresh-to-dried ratio).

You may also see a recipe that calls for an item you don't like. You can omit this ingredient altogether, or replace it with something similar.

I want you to view the recipes as inspiration and not the law. I hope you will try to get creative and put your own stank on my recipes (or, as we say in the South, "put yo foot in the recipes")!

As far as kitchen tools, there is nothing that bothers me more than gadgets with only one purpose, as they tend to take up too much kitchen space. I live in a studio apartment, so I know a thing or two about not having any space! With this in mind, I also made sure to include recipes that don't require you to have specialized equipment.

These are some basic kitchen items that are multi-functional and will have you throwing down in the kitchen and through this book in no time:

✓ a vegetable peeler

- ✓ a good blender (one with multi-speeds and a plug on top works well, but any blender that you have access to is a good start)
- ✓ a spiralizer that turns vegetables into noodles (optional; although Bed, Bath & Beyond has a little $15 one, which is what I use)
- ✓ a seasoned cast iron skillet (a well-oiled cast iron)
- ✓ a wire whisk
- ✓ a fine strainer
- ✓ tongs
- ✓ a kitchen thermometer (optional, if you don't have one, a small spoon will do to test the heat. With the small spoon, scoop out some of the batter and drop it into the hot oil. If it starts to float to the top you are in good shape)

Now let's get the cooking started…

This section is mainly for anyone who needs help or inspiration to get started on their journey towards plant-based eating and vegan living. If you are already a seasoned vegan, do check out the sauces and marinades in the following section, as well as the recipes, which are ones everyone will enjoy!

Sauces and Marinades

These basic sauces and marinades will get you started on your Southern-style plant based journey. You will need many of the following sauces and marinades for many of the recipes in this chapter, as well as the next one. Therefore, this is a good place to bookmark, since you can also refer to this specific section to add a little sumthang sumthang to your dishes once you feel ready to experiment on your own.

I refer to some of them as 'mother sauces' because you can use them as the base for other recipes throughout the book. I recommend making extra or keeping some on hand because it will make things much easier (and tastier!) when planning meals during the week.

Sauces

- *Basic Vegan Aioli (Mayo)*
- *Basic Cashew Cream*
- *Quick, Creamy Cashew Cheese*
- *Creamy Red Pepper Top Dip*
- *Black Pepper Mushroom Gravy*
- *Buffalo Sauce*

Basic Vegan Aioli (Mayo)

This is a super-easy recipe to make! Once you have this basic 'mother sauce' in stock, you can use it as a base for other sauces, like chipotle mayo. You can also use it as the base for things like sweet potato salad. This sauce stores really well in the fridge, and can even be frozen. If you need to defrost it, place the container in the back of your refrigerator for a few hours. You can also defrost it by placing the frozen mayo container for a few hours in a larger container, filled with cold water, in the sink.

Makes: ½ to 1 quart

Ingredients

1 block of silken or medium-firm tofu
1 cup of olive or canola oil
2 tablespoons of Dijon mustard
1 peeled garlic clove
¼ cup of lemon juice
1 teaspoon of salt
½ teaspoon of pepper
¼ teaspoon of cayenne pepper (optional)

Directions

1. Pour the lemon juice into the blender.

2. Add all of the remaining ingredients, EXCEPT for the oil, and blend until completely smooth.

3. Turn the blender down to a low speed. Unplug the top on the blender pitcher, then turn it back on to slowly drizzle in the oil until it has a thick, creamy mayo consistency.

Basic Cashew Cream

As with the aioli, this cashew cream is a base for other kinds of creamy sauces and dishes you'll find throughout this book. The difference between this and the aioli is that this one is soy-free, as well as oil-free— but does contain nuts. You can start with this sauce and experiment with different flavors to make your own dips and creams.

Makes: 2 to 4 cups

Ingredients

2 cups of raw cashews*
Enough water to cover the cashews in the blender

*As with other foods, when possible, try to buy fair trade cashews since they help workers earn a fair wage and provide better working conditions for them as well.

Directions

1. In a medium or large saucepan, boil the cashews in equal parts water until fully tender (about 15 to 20 minutes).

2. Drain the water in a strainer and run cold water over the cashews.

3. Place the cashews in a blender. Add enough fresh water to cover the top of the cashews.

4. Blend at a medium speed until it is completely velvety smooth without any chunks left.

5. Use now, or store this in the fridge for about 2-3 days.

Quick, Creamy Cashew Cheese

Makes: 1 cup

Ingredients

1 cup of **Basic Cashew Cream** (See page 42)
1 to 1 ½ tablespoons of apple cider vinegar
2 tablespoons of nutritional yeast
2 teaspoons of sea salt
1 teaspoon of garlic powder

Directions

1. In a medium-sized bowl, whisk all of the ingredients together.

2. Taste it! If it isn't cheesy enough for you, add more nutritional yeast. If it is too tangy, add ½ teaspoon more of sea salt. If it is too salty for your preference, thin it out with 2 tablespoons of water.

3. Store in the fridge and use within 2-3 days.

Creamy Red Pepper Top Dip

Makes: 1 ½ cups

Ingredients

1 cup of pepper scraps
½ cup of **Basic Cashew Cream** (See page 42)
1-2 teaspoons of salt
2 teaspoons of apple cider vinegar
1 teaspoon of pepper
½ teaspoon of cayenne pepper

Directions

1. Add all of the ingredients **EXCEPT** the cashew cream into the blender, and pulse them on a medium speed until they're fully broken (about 30-45 seconds).

2. Add the cashew cream and blend until you have a "red" (depending on the color of peppers you used), creamy spread.

3. Enjoy with homemade chips or fresh, raw vegetables.

Black Pepper Mushroom Gravy

Makes: 1 cup

Ingredients

1 cup of flour
¼ cup of olive oil (can sub with mild-flavor vegetable oil) + 1 tablespoon of olive oil
2 teaspoons of black pepper
1 teaspoon of salt
1 teaspoon of garlic powder
½ cup of diced onion
½ cup of chopped mushroom scraps or gills left over from other dishes
½ to 1 cup of vegetable stock

Directions

1. In a large skillet over medium heat, add 1 tablespoon of olive oil and sauté the mushroom scraps and onions until they have browned.

2. Pour in the flour; then, slowly pour in the remaining olive oil. As it starts to clump and form a "roux," turn down the heat slightly.

3. Whisk in the vegetable stock ¼ of a cup at a time. Whisk constantly in order to thin out the roux. Continue to pour in more stock until you reach the desired consistency of your gravy (I prefer a thinner, more uniform gravy that isn't very lumpy).

4. Add the salt, pepper, and garlic powder. Bring the heat down to low until you are ready to serve.

Buffalo Sauce

Makes: ½ cup

Ingredients

1 6- or 8-ounce bottle of Louisiana-style or Frank's Hot Sauce
¼ to ½ cup of melted vegan butter
½ teaspoon of cayenne pepper
1 teaspoon of garlic powder

Directions

1. In a medium saucepan over medium heat, melt the vegan butter (start with ¼ cup and adjust, if necessary).

2. Whisk in the other ingredients. The sauce should be a light orange color. If it is too thin and velvety, add the last ¼ cup of butter.

3. This can be stored in an airtight container in the fridge for 2-3 days.

Marinades

- *Eggy Marinade*
- *Faux Fish Marinade*
- *That Ain't NO Hog, Tho: Stanley B Pork Marinade*
- *Tastes Like Chicken Marinade*
- *Achin' for Steakin' Marinade*

Eggy Marinade

Makes: 1 cup

Ingredients

1 cup of olive, grapeseed or other mild, plant-based oil (except coconut oil)
1 tablespoon of apple cider vinegar
1 tablespoon of ground turmeric
1 tablespoon of garlic powder
1 tablespoon of nutritional yeast
2 teaspoons of sea salt
1 teaspoon of black pepper
1 teaspoon of black salt/kala namak (adds that pungent eggy/sulfuric taste)

Directions

1. Whisk all of the marinade ingredients together in a large bowl, *in the following order:* spices, apple cider vinegar, plant-based oil.

2. Use now or store in an airtight container in the fridge for 2-4 weeks.

Faux Fish Marinade

This recipe duplicates the essence of fish and seafood. You can use this on tofu, shiitake, and especially oyster mushrooms!

Makes: 1 cup

Ingredients

1 cup of olive or grapeseed oil
2 tablespoons of lemon juice (or a mild, white vinegar)
2 tablespoons of dulse* or kelp** flakes
2 teaspoons of old bay spice or other seafood spice blend***
2 teaspoons of thyme
1 teaspoon of black pepper
1 teaspoon of garlic powder
1 teaspoon of sea salt

*Dulse is a type of algae or sea vegetable. You can use dulse flakes to give food a seafood taste. The light purple or green flakes often come in a shaker and can be found in the spices or Asian food section of grocery stores.

**Kelp is another type of algae that can be found as sheets or flakes as used for the same reason as dulse.

***You can also make your own seafood blend by combining 2 tablespoons of ground bay leaves, 1 tablespoon of celery salt, 1 teaspoon black pepper, 1 teaspoon paprika, 1 teaspoon of all spice, 1 teaspoon ground cloves, and 1 teaspoon of crushed red pepper flakes.

Directions

1. Starting with the spices first, then the lemon juice/vinegar and lastly oil whisk together all the marinade ingredients in a large bowl.

2. Store in an airtight container in the fridge and use within 2-3 days.

That Ain't NO Hog, Tho: Stanley B Pork Marinade

My step-dad grew up in farm country in the central Texas town of Marlin, eating typically pork-centered meals. Although I haven't been able to get him to fully embrace plant-based eating (yet), whenever I am in Texas and make my plant-based bacon with this marinade, he's definitely a believer— "Even if it ain't no hog, tho!"

This recipe is great for tempeh bacon!

Makes: 1 cup

Ingredients

1 cup of olive oil
2 tablespoons of apple cider vinegar
2 tablespoons of nutritional yeast
1 teaspoon of liquid smoke (icing on the cake that gives it that smoky, bacony flavor)
1 teaspoon of black pepper
1 teaspoon of smoked paprika
1 tablespoon of sea salt
2 teaspoon of peanut butter
2 teaspoons of molasses (iron boost that also balances flavors!)

Directions

1. Starting with the spices first, then the liquids, then peanut butter, and lastly, the oil, whisk all the ingredients together in a large bowl.

2. Store in an airtight container in the fridge and use up to 2-3 days.

Tastes Like Chicken Marinade

This marinade is great on tofu, seitan, and wild mushrooms.

Makes: 1 cup

Ingredients

1 cup of olive oil
2 tablespoons of white or apple cider vinegar
2 tablespoons of nutritional yeast
2 tablespoons of poultry seasoning
2 teaspoons of thyme
1 teaspoon of garlic powder
1 teaspoon of sea salt
1 teaspoon of black pepper

Directions

1. Starting with the spices first, then the vinegar, and lastly, the oil, whisk together all the marinade ingredients in a large bowl.

2. Store in an airtight container in the fridge and eat it up in 2-3 days.

Achin' for Steakin' Marinade

This great for portabella mushroom steaks or beet filet mignon!

Makes: 1 cup

Ingredients

1 cup of olive or grapeseed oil
2 tablespoons of apple cider vinegar
1 tablespoon of cumin
2 teaspoons of garlic of powder
½ teaspoon of liquid smoke
2 teaspoons of black pepper
2 teaspoons of steak seasoning
1 teaspoon of sea salt
1 tablespoon of nutritional yeast
1 teaspoon of molasses

Directions

1. Starting with the spices first, then the vinegar and, lastly, the oil, whisk together all the marinade ingredients in a large bowl.

2. Store in an airtight container in the fridge and use within 2-3 days.

Jumpstart Week One

Are you ready to jump in, plant-based style?

For my newbies, let's get you started with a week-long eating plan— including recipes so easy that you will get this plant-based eating down so quickly, you will be a pro by Week Two and be ready to build your own meal plan (See Page 90).

Jumpstart Week One Meals

	Breakfast	Lunch	Dinner
Monday	Tex-Mex Breakfast Bowl	Blanny Blan's Grilled Toficken Tahini Caesar Salad	Faux Pork Pineapple Fried Rice Boat
Tuesday	'Egg' Muffin Sandwich	Roasted Squash Bowl	Cam's Burger Helper
Wednesday	Pass Tha Greens Smoothie	Naw Egg Salad	Southern Fried Cauli-Chicken Soul Bowl
Thursday	Sweet Potato Toast with Smoky Apple Nut Butter	Sweet Potato Steaks	Margherita Pizza
Friday	Oat to Joy Smoothie	Sassy Cat's Black Bean Tostadas with Roasted Corn Salsa	Taste Like Thanksgiving Stuffed Butternut Squash
Saturday	Silky, Cheesy Scram-On-The-Go Pocket	'Meatloaf' Stuffed Large Portobello Caps	Cajun Pulled Artichoke 'Chicken' with Dirty Rice
Sunday	Sweet Southern Boy Stuffed, Baked Pocket	Taco Salad	Jerk Cauliflower Chicken Wings

Here's a quick list of what you will need to follow along with week one:

Grocery List

1 canister of oatmeal
1 package of English Muffin
1 jar of nut butter (for example, peanut butter or almond butter)
1 jar of jam or fruit preserves
3-4 bananas
1 package of vegan deli-style meat (optional)
4 blocks of firm or extra firm tofu

2 quarts of non-dairy milk
1 avocado
4 tomatoes
2 bell peppers
2 large onions
2 8oz or larger packs of tempeh
6 large sweet potatoes
1 date (optional; you can use agave syrup, sugar, or other types of sweeteners)
1 bunch of cilantro
3 pizza doughs (pre-made store-bought dough, not pizza crust)
1 package of cashew for cheese (you can also use a pre-made vegan cheese instead if you prefer)
1 container of tahini sauce
3 packs of small mushrooms (like button mushrooms, which are also known as cremini mushrooms)
1 lemon
1 lime
1 small jar of capers
1 can of olives
1 can of "Rotel" tomato and onion blend, or "sofrito"
2 bunches of spinach or kale (or a combination of both)
1 package of shredded lettuce or a head of iceberg
1 bunch or a sturdy green like collards or mustard greens
2 small squashes
1 32-ounce package of rice
1 package of tortillas
1 can of black beans
1 jar of vegan mayo
2 jalapeños
1 can of refried beans
2 large tostada shells or a box of crispy taco shells
4 large portabella mushroom caps
2 small tins of tomato paste
1 container of vegan cream cheese
1 whole pineapple or 1 can of pineapple chunks in water not syrup
1 package of elbow macaroni or pasta
1 package of tempeh or beef-less crumbles
1 sweet potato or canned purée
1 head of cauliflower
1 package 3-5 lb bag of flour
1 bunch of fresh or dried basil
4-6 slices of bread
1 large butternut squash
1 package of cranberries or pomegranate
1 package of golden raisins

Be sure to also stock up on these:

Pantry Staples

Nutritional yeast
Cumin
Salt
Black pepper
Black salt or Himalayan salt
Apple cider vinegar
Olive oil
Balsamic vinegar
Sugar (or another type of sweetener)

Molasses
Seasoning salt or poultry seasoning
Dried thyme
Dried sage
Turmeric
Garlic powder
Liquid smoke*
Maple syrup

*Liquid smoke can be found for about $3 or less in the BBQ sauce section of grocery stores. It helps give marinades and other foods a mesquite, smoky flavor.

Week One: Breakfasts

Tex-Mex Breakfast Bowl

Makes: 1 to 2 servings

Ingredients

¾ cup of cooked oatmeal
½ cup of diced, firm tofu
¼ cup of **Eggy Marinade** (See Page 49)
¼ cup of diced tomato
¼ cup of diced red onion (any onion works; red ones are just milder)
1 minced jalapeño
2 tablespoons of minced cilantro
½ cup of spinach (or your preferred dark, leafy green)
1 teaspoon of garlic salt
1 tablespoon of olive oil or cooking spray
¼ of an avocado, sliced or diced (you can store the rest of the avocado in the fridge by leaving the large pit in and wrapping it tightly with plastic wrap; consume within 1-2 days as it will turn brown)

Directions

1. Pour the EGG Marinade into a small bowl and whisk it with a fork or a whisk to reconstitute it.

2. Dice the tofu and add it to the marinade. Set aside.

3. Cook the oatmeal according to the directions. While oatmeal is cooking, dice all the vegetables.

4. Heat the tablespoon of olive oil in a medium-sized skillet over medium heat. Add the marinade tofu-egg and sauté until slightly golden (about 3-5 minutes). Remove from heat.

5. Add the spinach to the same skillet you used for the tofu-egg. Sprinkle on the garlic salt. Using tongs or a fork, lightly sauté for 1-2 minutes.

6. To assemble bowl, place the oatmeal on the bottom of a cereal bowl. Next, top with the spinach. Place a row of the tofu-egg on the bed of sautéed spinach. Garnish the bowl with the diced tomato, onion, jalapeño, avocado and cilantro.

7. Enjoy with your favorite hot sauce.

'Egg' Muffin Sandwich

Makes: 2 to 4 sandwiches

Ingredients

1 block of firm tofu
½ cup of **Eggy Marinade** (See Page 49)
2-4 toasted English muffins (depending on how many sandwiches you want to make)
1 medium-sized tomato, cut into thick slices
½ tablespoon of olive oil or cooking spray
2-4 tablespoons of your favorite jam, or my **Plum Jam** (See Page 124)
2-4 slices of **Tempeh Bacon** (See Page 107) or your favorite vegan deli-style meat (optional)

Directions

1. Pour the **Eggy Marinade** into a medium or large bowl. Whisk with a fork or a whisk if the marinade has separated.

2. Slice the block of tofu in half, lengthwise. Slice the halves in half lengthwise if you are making more than 2 sandwiches.

3. Use a small, glass, circular cookie cutter or a measuring cup to punch out the tofu blocks into rounds. Place the rounds into the marinade, making sure to fully drench each side.

4. Heat the olive oil in a medium or large skillet over medium heat. Place the "egg" rounds in the skillet, two at a time, and press down with a slotted spatula to sear. Cook for 2-3 minutes on each side. Remove from heat and use this same skillet to hit vegan "meat," if you are using any.

5. Toast the English muffins.

6. Assemble the sandwiches by smearing the jam onto each half of the muffin. On the bottom half, place an egg patty. Drizzle 1 teaspoon of the marinade on the patty to simulate a yolk. Top the egg patty with a thick tomato slice (and vegan "meat," if desired).

7. Enjoy right away!

Pass Tha Greens Smoothie

Makes: 2 smoothies

Ingredients

1 banana
1 ½ cup of non-dairy milk (try one fortified with B12!)
2-3 cups of spinach, or another fresh green, such as kale
1 cup of ice
1 tablespoon of nut butter, such as peanut butter
1 scoop of vanilla or chocolate vegan protein powder **OR** ¼ cup of plain, dried, old-fashioned oats (NOT steel cut)

Directions

1. Pour the non-dairy milk into the blender.

2. Add the banana, protein powder, spinach, peanut butter, and ice, in that order.

3. Turn the blender on to its lowest speed and blend for a few seconds.

4. Incrementally increase the speed and blend until it is smooth and you have reached your desired texture.

5. Taste and sweeten as needed.

6. Serve immediately.

Sweet Potato Toast with Smoky Apple Nut Butter

This is a fast and inexpensive breakfast idea. Play around with other combinations, like vegan cream cheese and capers, guacamole and tomatoes, or even my **Savory Scram** (See Page 113)!

Makes: 4 to 8 toasts

Ingredients

1-2 medium-sized, fresh sweet potatoes or yams (1 will make about 4 pieces of toast)
¼ cup of your favorite nut butter, such as peanut butter
4 tablespoons of apple jam (store-bought; just make sure it is vegan!)
1 teaspoon of liquid smoke
2 tablespoons of fresh, chopped nuts (optional)

Directions

1. In a small- or medium-sized bowl, whisk together the jam, liquid smoke, and nut butter. Set aside.

2. Wash the sweet potatoes and slice them into ¼-inch thick slices. Turn your toaster to its highest setting and place a potato slice into each opening. Toast the sweet potato until soft, but not completely mushy. The number of cycles this will take will depend on your toaster, so test for firmness at the end of each toasting cycle.

3. Smear a generous amount of nut butter spread on each sweet potato toast. Top with the chopped nuts, if using.

Oat to Joy Smoothie

Makes: 2 smoothies

Ingredients

1 cup of coconut milk
¼ cup of uncooked oats
1 banana
2 tablespoons of cocoa powder (or 1 scoop of chocolate vegan protein powder)
1 pitted date (or other sweeter such as 1 tablespoon of agave, sugar, or maple syrup)
1 cup of ice cubes

Directions

1. Place the coconut milk into the blender.

2. Add all of the remaining ingredients.

3. Turn the blender to its lowest speed and blend for 10-15 seconds.

4. Incrementally increase the blender speed and blend until you have reached your preferred texture.

5. Enjoy immediately.

Stuffed, Baked Breakfast Pockets

These next two breakfast-pocket recipes are great for weekends when you have more time or want to host brunches. You can also make these ahead of time and freeze them for quick weekday or on-the-go breakfasts. Simply reheat them in the oven or microwave.

Silky, Cheesy Scram-On-The-Go Pocket

Makes: 2 large pockets*

*Divide the dough into smaller pieces for smaller pockets.

Ingredients

1 pre-made vegan pizza dough
2 cups of **Savory Scram** (See Page 113)
¼ cup **Quick, Creamy Cashew Cheese** (See Page 43), or your favorite store-bought
   vegan cheese
¼ cup of diced tomato
2 tablespoons of minced cilantro for garnish (once the pockets are fully cooked)
2 tablespoons + 2 teaspoons of olive oil
½ cup of flour for the surface

Directions

1. Use a rubber spatula to grease the inside of a large bowl with 1 tablespoon of olive oil. Remove the dough from its wrapper and place it in the bowl. Let the dough set out at room temperature for 30 minutes.

2. Preheat the oven to 475 °F. In a medium or large skillet, heat 1 tablespoon of olive oil. Sauté the **Savory Scram** in the skillet for 2-3 minutes. Set aside.

3. Flour a clean kitchen surface. Remove the dough from the bowl and divide it into two equal pieces. Using a floured rolling pin, roll out the dough.

4. Smear half of the **Creamy Cashew Cheese** along one half of each piece of dough. Using a large spoon, scoop a generous amount of the scram onto the cheese. Sprinkle the tomatoes on top of the scram.

5. Fold the topping-less half of the dough over the half with toppings, calzone-style. Use your fingers to press the edges close. Repeat this with the remaining dough and toppings.

6. Drizzle an additional teaspoon of olive oil on to the top of each pocket. Using a small knife, cut two slits on top each pocket to *vent* (so that the inside cooks thoroughly).

7. Place the pockets on a well-oiled baking sheet or a pizza stone. Bake them in the oven for 15- 20 minutes, or until golden brown. Garnish with cilantro.

8. Eat right away or freeze (after they have cooled) in freezer-safe bags.

Sweet Southern Boy Stuffed, Baked Pocket

Makes: 2 large pockets*

*Divide the dough into smaller pieces for smaller pockets.

Ingredients

1 package of pre-made vegan pizza dough
¼ cup of your favorite nut butter
1 cup of **Tempeh Bacon** (See Page 107), or your favorite store-bought vegan bacon
1 sliced banana
2 tablespoons + 2 teaspoons of olive oil
½ cup of flour for the surface

Directions

1. Use a rubber spatula to grease the inside of a large bowl with 1 tablespoon of olive oil. Remove the dough from its wrapper and place it in the bowl. Let the dough set out at room temperature for 30 minutes.

2. Preheat the oven to 475°F. In a medium or large skillet, heat 1 tablespoon of olive oil. Sauté the **Tempeh Bacon** in the skillet for 2-3 minutes. Set aside.

3. Flour a clean kitchen surface. Remove the dough from the bowl and divide it into two equal pieces. Using a floured rolling pin, roll out the dough.

4. Smear half of the nut butter along one half of each piece of dough. Lay some of the banana slices on top of the nut butter. Crumble the tempeh bacon and sprinkle it over the banana slices and nut butter.

5. Fold the topping-less half of the dough over the half with toppings, calzone-style. Use your fingers to press the edges close. Repeat this with the remaining dough and toppings.

6. Drizzle an additional teaspoon of olive oil on to the top of each pocket. Using a small knife, cut two slits on the top each pocket to *vent* (so that the inside cooks thoroughly).

7. Place the pockets on a well-oiled baking sheet or a pizza stone. Bake in the oven for 15- 20 minutes, or until golden brown.

8. Eat right away or freeze (after they have cooled) in freezer-safe bags.

Week One: Lunch

Blanny Blan's Grilled Toficken Tahini Caesar Salad

My best friend, Blanny, and I have our own little "slanguage" in which we blend words to create new ones, and you just learned two of 'em! His real name is Danny, but I changed it to Blanny during one adventurous college day over twelve years ago (nope, not gonna tell!). The second is "Toficken," which is Blanny's word for tofu-chicken. This recipe is my ode to Blanny.

Makes: 1 large salad

Ingredients

½ cup of **Tastes Like Chicken Marinade** (See Page 52),
1 block of extra firm tofu
3 cups of chopped kale (or your preferred type of lettuce)
1 tablespoon of olive oil
¼ cup of vegan croutons*

Ingredients for Caesar Dressing:

½ cup of tahini sauce
2 tablespoons of lemon juice
2 tablespoons of capers (minced)
1 teaspoon of garlic salt (or 1 tsp of garlic powder + 1 teaspoon of salt)
1 teaspoon of pepper
¼-½ cup of water if desired, to thin out the dressing

*You can make your own by dicing stale bread, sprinkling 1 teaspoon of garlic salt on the dices, drizzling 2 tablespoons of olive oil over them, and baking them at 400°F for about 20 minutes.

Directions

1. Wrap the block of tofu in a napkin and place it on a plate. Place a heavy book or cast-iron pan on the tofu block to press it, which will squeeze out any excess water.

2. While the tofu is pressing, make the Caesar dressing. Take all the dressing ingredients (tahini sauce, lemon juice, minced capers, garlic salt, and pepper) EXCEPT the water and whisk them together in a medium or large bowl. If it is too thick for your preference, thin it out with water, ¼ cup at a time. Set aside.

3. Heat 1 tablespoon of olive oil in a cast iron pan.

4. Slice the tofu into ¼-inch or ½-inch steaks. If you want it to have grilled marks, *score* the tofu slices (make cross-hatch slits in an "X" pattern, but do not cut through it). Place the toficken steaks in a bowl of the **Tastes Like Chicken Marinade**. Fully drench the steaks, making sure each side is fully coated.

5. Place the steaks in the hot cast iron skillet, pressing down to sear them. Let them stick for about 1-2 minutes so they can get that nice, nutty char. Flip over and repeat on the other side.

6. Place the chopped greens in a large bowl. Drizzle ¼ cup of the tahini dressing over the greens. Massage the dressing into the greens with your hands or toss the salad with tongs.

7. Put the greens in a large bowl (or divide into two bowls, if sharing) Top with a grilled toficken steak. Garnish with croutons.

8. The remaining dressing can be stored in a sealed container in the fridge for about 2-3 days.

Roasted Squash Bowl

Makes: 1 to 2 bowls

Ingredients

1-2 small autumn squashes, such as "Delicata"*
2 cups of cooked brown rice
½ cup of a fresh green such as arugula (any other dark green you can find works too)
¼ cup of golden raisins
¼ of olive oil
2 teaspoons of thyme
2 teaspoons of turmeric
2 teaspoons of sea salt
1 teaspoon of black pepper
3 tablespoons of balsamic vinaigrette or your favorite vegan salad dressing

*If you can't find a fresh one, you can use a 12-16-ounce package of another fresh, pre-cut squash, such as butternut squash chunks, in the produce section.

Directions

1. Preheat the oven to 400°F.

2. Wash the squash off if it still has skin on it. Slice it lengthwise and scoop out the seeds.

3. Slice the deseeded squash into half-rings. Set aside.

4. In a large- or medium-sized bowl, add the olive oil, 1 teaspoon of thyme, all of the turmeric, 1 teaspoon of salt and all of the pepper. Whisk them together.

5. Add the squash rings (or chunks of pre-cut squash) into the marinade and toss with a large spoon to fully coat the squash.

6. Place the squash on a baking sheet and bake until tender (15-20 minutes).

7. While the squash is roasting, reheat the rice if it isn't warm already.

8. To assemble the bowl, place the cooked rice at the bottom of your serving bowl (can be split into two bowls if sharing, using 1 cup for each). Next, add a generous handful of greens on top of the rice (the leftover heat from the rice will gently wilt the greens, adding more depth of flavor!). Place the squash rings/chunks on top of the bed of greens. Garnish with the raisins.

9. Drizzle the balsamic vinaigrette on top if you are eating right away. If you are packing this dish to take to work for lunch, then add the salad dressing when you are ready to eat it.

Naw Egg Salad

Makes: 2 to 4 servings

Ingredients

1 block of firm tofu (diced)
¼ cup of diced celery (save the leaves from the stalks if you have them)
½ cup of diced red onion
¼ cup of bell pepper (diced)
½ cup fresh diced tomato
2 tablespoons of mustard
2 teaspoon of apple cider vinegar or distilled vinegar
2 teaspoons of garlic salt
1 teaspoon of black salt
1 teaspoon of black pepper
1 teaspoon of turmeric
2 tablespoons of minced celery leaves, for garnish (optional, but they add a nice freshness!)
⅓ cup of store-bought vegan mayo or my **Basic Vegan Aioli (Mayo)** (See Page 41) (if you prefer a creamier salad, add an additional 2 tablespoon of mayo)

Directions

1. Cut the tofu into small, die-shaped pieces. Place half of it in a small bowl. Sprinkle on the turmeric, black salt and 1 teaspoon of apple cider vinegar. (This is the yolk part of the "egg" salad.) Mix with a spoon and set aside.

2. Dice all of the vegetables and set them aside.

3. In a large bowl, whisk the garlic salt, pepper, vegan mayo, mustard, and remaining vinegar together.

4. Add the vegetables and all of the tofu, and mix it all together with a large spoon.

5. Enjoy on toast, over mixed greens, or with large romaine leaves as lettuce wraps.

Tip: Make extra to save for a quick salad lunch for a few days!

Sweet Potato Steaks

Makes: 4 to 6 steaks

Ingredients

2 medium-to-large sweet potatoes
½ cup of **Achin' for Steakin' Marinade** (See Page 53)
1 tablespoon of olive oil or cooking spray to prevent the steaks from sticking

Directions

1. Preheat oven to 400°F.

2. Wash the sweet potatoes, but keep the skin on for extra fiber!

3. Slice the potatoes into ¼-inch or ½-inch "steaks."

4. Pour the marinade into a large bowl and whisk if it has separated. Add the steaks to the marinade and toss them to coat each side.

5. Spray a cooking sheet or spread olive oil over it with a spatula so that it is fully coated. Add the steaks, leaving space in between them so they don't touch. Bake in the oven for 12-15 minutes on each side (check on them after about 20 minutes!). You want them slightly "al dente," but not mushy.

6. Drizzle an extra tablespoon of oil on top (optional).

Sassy Cat's Black Bean Tostadas with Roasted Corn Salsa

Born two and half years after me, my little sister Cathy has been charting her own path through life. While I've spent much of my adulthood as a pseudo-drifter bouncing from coast to coast, she's been holding it down for the Hill girls in Texas. Two years ago, she followed my steps and began a plant-based journey of her own. This dish is for you, Seester (her text nickname for me), based on your favorite food: black bean tacos!

Makes: 4 tostadas

Ingredients

1 can of black beans, cooked
4 crispy tostada shells
1 red bell pepper
1 jalapeño (Deseed if you aren't a fan of heat, but then they won't be as sassy!)
1 cup of chopped or shredded lettuce (iceberg to keep it traditional)
1 ½ tablespoon of taco seasoning
½ red onion sliced into thin rings
⅓ cup of distilled vinegar
2 tablespoons of sugar
½ cup of boiling water
2 teaspoons of salt
1 sliced avocado, for garnish (optional)

Ingredients for Corn Salsa:

1 can of corn
1 small tomato, diced
¼ cup of minced cilantro (or 1 teaspoon of coriander powder)
1 tablespoon cooking oil
½ cup of diced onion
1 teaspoon of sea salt
Juice of 1 lime

Directions

1. Preheat your oven's broiler. While the broiler is heating, cook the beans in a medium saucepan.

2. Drain the liquid from the can of corn and place the corn in a bowl. Pour oil and salt over the corn and toss it with a spoon.

3. Pour the corn into a small roasting pan or cast-iron skillet and place it in the broiler. Stay close, because they can get *incinerated* in only 4 minutes! Once they are

charred (when the kernel edges become nutty or black), it is ready. Remove the pan from the oven and turn off the broiler.

4. Place the roasted corn in a bowl and add all of the other salsa ingredients (tomato, minced cilantro or coriander powder, oil, onion, sea salt, and lime juice). Toss everything with a spoon and set it aside.

5. In a small saucepan or boiler, boil the ½ cup of water. Remove from heat.

6. Pour the boiling water in a small bowl and add the sugar, vinegar, and 2 teaspoons of salt. Whisk them together for a quick pickle by adding red onions into the solution.

7. In a blender, add the cooked black beans, taco seasoning, jalapeño, and red bell pepper. Blend until it forms a nice paste.

8. To assemble, smear a generous amount of the paste onto each tostada shell. Next, sprinkle the shells with shredded lettuce and top them with roasted corn salsa. Sprinkle the pickled red onions on top for a tangy topper that balances all the flavors.

9. Garnish with avocado slices, if desired.

"Meatloaf"-Stuffed Large Portobello Caps

Makes: 2 to 4 caps

Ingredients

2-4 large portabella mushroom caps, cleaned, with the gills removed
1 thin can of tomato paste
1 8-12-ounce package of tempeh
½ cup of small diced onion
¼ cup of small diced green bell pepper
2 chopped garlic cloves or 1 teaspoon of garlic powder
1 tablespoon of molasses
1 teaspoon of dried or fresh thyme
2 tablespoons olive oil
1 tablespoon of salt
1 teaspoon of black pepper
2 teaspoons of cumin
2 cups of water (to boil)

Directions

1. Preheat oven to 375°F. Bring 2 cups of water to boil.

2. Crumble the tempeh into meaty chunks on a cutting board. Once the water reaches a rolling boil, add the crumbled tempeh to the pot and boil for about 3 minutes. Drain the tempeh in a mesh strainer or colander and set aside.

3. Heat 1 tablespoon of olive oil into a large skillet on medium heat. Add the diced onion, bell pepper, and fresh garlic (if using) and sauté for about 3-5 minutes, until onions are translucent.

4. Add the tempeh to the skillet, followed by the remaining spices and molasses. Sauté for 3-5 minutes, until brown.

5. Add a generous spoonful of tomato paste into the skillet of tempeh. Mix to fully incorporate the paste and remove from the heat.

6. Using a large spoon, take a spoonful of the sautéed tempeh and fill each mushroom cap. Drizzle the remaining olive oil on the bottom of a baking sheet to prevent the caps from sticking. Place the stuffed caps onto the baking sheets.

7. Using a rubber spatula or large butter knife, smear the remaining tomato paste onto the top of each stuffed mushroom cap (like frosting a cake). Bake for 20-25 minutes, until tender.

8. Enjoy right away, or pack for tomorrow's lunch.

Taco Salad

Makes: 1 large salad*

*This recipe makes 1 large salad if you use a taco shell bowl. If you use boxed shells, then this will make 2 salads.

Ingredients

1 large taco shell/tostada to use as the salad bowl (if you can't find one that big, just get a few crispy taco shells from a box)
1 can of vegan refried beans (look out for lard as an ingredient, which is not vegan!)
2 teaspoons of garlic powder
2 teaspoons of salt
1 can of "Rotel"-style tomato-and-diced-onion mix (or ½ cup of store-bought sofrito, which is usually found in the "ethnic" aisle at the grocery store)
¼ cup of store-bought vegan cream cheese mixed with 1 tablespoon of apple cider vinegar and 1 tablespoon of nutritional yeast; or use ½ cup of my **Quick, Creamy Cashew Cheese** (See Page 43)
2-3 cups of shredded or chopped lettuce, such as iceberg or romaine
1 diced jalapeño
2 tablespoons of sliced black or green olives

Directions

1. In a medium saucepan, cook the refried beans with the salt and garlic powder.

2. Whisk the vegan cream cheese, vinegar, and nutritional yeast together and set aside (skip this step if using cashew cheese).

3. Drain the can of "Rotel" tomato mix (if using).

4. If using large tostada bowl, sprinkle a small handful of the shredded lettuce onto the bottom of the shell. This is to prevent the shell from getting soggy. If you are using a regular bowl, place a handful of lettuce on the bottom of the bowl.

5. Place a generous amount of beans onto the lettuce. Top the beans with the "Rotel" or "sofrito." Use a large spoon to drop a dollop of the cheese on top of the tomato.

6. Sprinkle the olives and jalapeños throughout the top layer of the salad. If using the taco shells from the box, crumble the shell over the salad as a crunchy crouton.

Week One: Dinner

Faux Pork Pineapple Fried Rice Boat

Makes: 2 boats

Ingredients

½ cup of diced pineapple from a whole pineapple (you can use the pineapple as an
    interesting serving bowl but if you don't feel comfortable with cutting a whole
    pineapple, then use a can of pineapple chunks)
½ cup of diced onion
¼ cup of diced bell pepper
1 cup of diced tofu
¼ cup of **That Ain't NO Hog, Tho: Stanley B Pork Marinade** (See Page 51)
2 cups of cooked brown rice (or your favorite rice)
2 tablespoons of olive oil
½ cup of pineapple juice from the fresh pineapple or the juice from the can
2 teaspoons of garlic salt
1 teaspoon of black pepper

Directions

1. Pour the **Marinade** into a small bowl. Dice the tofu and add it to the marinade. Toss with a spoon to let the tofu marinate. Set aside.

2. If you are using the whole pineapple, slice the pineapple in half lengthwise. Use a knife to remove the core that runs through the middle (while keeping the pineapple shell intact). It may be easier to remove the core by scooping out the pineapple flesh first and saving it in a separate bowl with the juice.

3. Use a strainer to separate the pineapple from the juice. Chop the pineapple flesh to use in the rice. Skip this step if you are using canned pineapple.

4. Heat the olive oil in a large skillet or wok over medium heat. Add the onion and bell pepper to the skillet and sauté until the onions turn translucent (about 3 minutes).

5. Add the diced tofu "pork" into the skillet of *aromatics* (the onions and peppers) and brown by stirring occasionally, for about 3 minutes, with a large spoon.

6. Add the cooked rice, garlic salt, and black pepper. Stir everything together to fully incorporate all of the ingredients. Let the rice stick to the pan for a couple of minutes before stirring further (this will brown the rice and give it a nice, nutty, roasted flavor).

7. Add the pineapple chunks and continue to stir. Reduce the heat and drizzle the pineapple juice to deglaze the pan. Cook for an additional 2-3 minutes.

8. If you are using the hollowed-out pineapples, scoop out the rice and fill each half with them.

9. Serve immediately.

Cam's Burger Helper

Makes: 2 to 4 servings

Growing up with a busy, working mom, Hamburger Helper made several appearances at my house throughout the week. It's filling, surprisingly flavorful (especially since it came from a box with a powder for seasoning) and easy to make. Although those box days are long gone, this plant-based take on it definitely brings back those warm, filling memories.

Ingredients

1 package of elbow macaroni (or other pasta shape you like, such as spirals or rotini)
1-2 8oz packages of tempeh, depending on how meaty you want it (you can also use 2-3 cups of store-bought ground beef-less crumbles)
2 tablespoons of olive oil

Ingredients for the Cheezy Sauce:

1 ½ cups of **Quick, Creamy Cashew Cheese** (See Page 43)
1 cooked sweet potato (or substitute with 1 cup of canned sweet potato, orange
   squash, or pumpkin)
1 teaspoon of garlic powder
1 teaspoon of salt and black pepper
⅓ cup of vegan milk (such as almond, coconut, or soy)

Ingredients for "Meat" Seasoning:

¼ cup of tomato paste
2 teaspoons of cumin
1 teaspoon of chili powder
2 teaspoons of garlic salt
1 tablespoon of balsamic vinegar
2 tablespoons of water to thin out
1 teaspoon of salt
1 teaspoon of black pepper

Directions

1. Cook the pasta, drain, and set aside.

2. To make Cheezy Sauce, pour the vegan milk into a blender. Add the remaining Cheezy Sauce ingredients (**Quick, Creamy Cashew Cheese**, sweet potato, garlic powder, salt, and pepper) to the blender and blend on a low to medium speed for 1-3 minutes until you have a uniform sauce. Set aside.

3. Heat 2 tablespoons of olive oil in a large skillet over medium heat. If you are using tempeh, season it with 1 teaspoon of salt and pepper, crumble it, and add it to the skillet. If you are using the store-bought beef-style meat, season it with 1 teaspoon of salt and pepper and then add it to the skillet. Sauté to brown by using a large spoon to stir and cook evenly for about 3-6 minutes.

4. Add all of the "meat" seasoning to a small bowl and whisk together. Pour the mixture over the "meat."

5. Add the cooked pasta to the large skillet of "meat." Pour the Cheezy Sauce into the skillet and mix well, thereby coating the entire dish. Simmer for 5-8 minutes, stirring occasionally, until some of the liquid has evaporated, but it still creamy.

6. Enjoy right away or freeze to eat later.

Southern Fried Cauli-Chicken Soul Bowl

Makes: 2 to 4 bowls

Ingredients

1 head of cauliflower or 1 bag of cauliflower florets
2 cups of flour
2 tablespoons of season salt or poultry seasoning
1 cup of vegan milk + 1 tablespoon of apple cider vinegar
2 cups vegetable oil for frying
1 bunch of collard greens (you *can* use canned, but what kind of Texan would I be if I
   didn't tell you how to do the real thang?)
1 teaspoon of distilled vinegar or apple cider vinegar
1 teaspoon of garlic salt
1 teaspoon of liquid smoke
2 tablespoon of olive oil or grapeseed oil
3 cups of cooked rice (use more if you are making more than 4 bowls)
2 diced yams or sweet potatoes
1 teaspoon of nutmeg

Directions

1. Preheat oven to 375°F.

2. Cut the sweet potato into a medium dice. Add the sweet potatoes to a medium-sized bowl. Pour the nutmeg onto the sweet potatoes, and drizzle 1 tablespoon of olive oil over them.

3. Toss the potatoes in the bowl using a large spoon, or, if you're a pro, toss them within the bowl itself!

4. Pour the potatoes on a well-oiled baking sheet and bake in the oven for 20-25 minutes, until tender.

5. While the potatoes are roasting, prepare the cauliflower for frying. First, remove the florets from the head if using and place on a cutting board. If using a bag of florets, just put them directly on the cutting board. Sprinkle ½ tablespoon of season salt over all the florets.

6. In a deep pot or fryer, pour in the cooking oil about 4 inches high (you should have enough to completely cover the top of the cauliflower). While the oil is getting to temperature (between 385°F and 400°F), set up your breading station.

7. Set up three bowls:

-add 1 cup of flour in the first bowl.
-the middle bowl should be filled with the cup of milk and vinegar mixture.
-the last bowl should be filled with 1 cup of flour mixed with the remaining
 tablespoon of season salt.

8. Once oil reaches temperature and it is bubbling, but not smoking, it is ready for frying. Dip a floret into the first bowl of flour. Next, dip it into the liquid bowl, and finally, the last bowl with the seasoned flour. Place in the fryer. Repeat this process with the remaining pieces, being careful not to overcrowd the pot.

9. Using tongs or a metal-slotted spoon, fry the florets until they are golden on each side and crispy (about 2-3 minutes). Place them on a plate lined with a paper towel.

10. Rinse off the fresh collard greens. Stack the leaves, 3-4 at a time, on top of each other and roll them up, cigar-style. Slice the greens into thin strips.*

11. Heat 1 tablespoon of olive oil in a large skillet over medium heat and add the collard greens. Then, add the garlic salt, vinegar, and liquid smoke. Sauté using tongs for 2-4 minutes, until they are wilted, but not soggy. Set aside.

12. To assemble the bowls, place a few generous scoops of cooked rice at the bottom of a bowl. Next, place a few spoonfuls of sweet potatoes in a row on top of the rice. Using tongs, place some greens next to the sweet potatoes. Lastly, top the bowl with a few florets of cauliflower chicken.

13. Enjoy with some Louisiana hot sauce on top (you know I keep some in my bag!).

*This style of chopping, which is normally done on herbs, is called *chiffonade* or ribbon-style, since the greens will be left looking like thin pieces of ribbon.

Margherita Pizza

Makes 1 pizza; 6-8 slices

Ingredients

1 package of pre-made pizza dough
2 slightly firm tomatoes, sliced
1 ½ cups of **Quick, Creamy Cashew Cheese** (See Page 43)
1 teaspoon of sea salt
1 black pepper
1 cup of fresh, chopped basil
2 tablespoons of olive oil
½ cup of flour

Directions

1. Using a rubber spatula, oil the sides of a large bowl with 1 tablespoon of olive oil. Remove the dough from its wrapper and place it in the bowl. Let it sit in the bowl at room temperature for 30 minutes.

2. Preheat the oven to 475°F. Slice the tomatoes into ¼-inch slices.

3. Remove the dough from the bowl. Punch out the pizza dough ball. Lay the dough on the floured surface and, using a floured rolling pin, roll out the pizza dough.

4. Stretch the dough onto a pizza stone or a large, flat sheet pan. Put the pan of dough in the oven for 3-5 minutes.

5. Remove the dough from the oven and, using a rubber spatula, spread the **Cashew Cheese** all over the dough's surface.

6. Place the tomato slices all over the surface of the pizza. Sprinkle the salt and pepper over the tomatoes. Garnish the pizza with half of the fresh basil.

7. Bake the pizza for 10-15 minutes, until the tomatoes wrinkle and the crust turns golden. Top the pizza with the remaining fresh basil.

8. Slice with a pizza cutter and serve.

Tastes Like Thanksgiving Stuffed Butternut Squash

Makes: 2 to 4 servings

Ingredients

1 large whole butternut squash
3 slices of bread, preferably stale and diced into chunks (I like to use the ends, which
   we call the "booty" in Texas!)
¼ cup of pomegranate seeds (dried or fresh cranberries will also work well)
¼ cup of diced onion and bell pepper
1 tablespoon of minced fresh thyme (or 2 teaspoons of dried thyme)
2 teaspoons of cumin
1 teaspoon of sea salt
1 teaspoon of minced fresh sage (or ½ teaspoon of ground sage powder)
1 tablespoon garlic salt
2 tablespoons of olive oil or grapeseed oil
1 teaspoon of black pepper
½ cup of water
1 tablespoon of sugar or your choice of sweetener

Directions

1. Preheat oven to 400°F. Wash the outside of the squash. Slice in half lengthwise with a very sharp knife. It is easiest to do this by first cutting off the tiny stem and then standing the squash up on its bottom. Place a napkin under the cutting board to prevent it from slipping. Then, starting from the top, where the stem was, press the knife through the squash from top to bottom.

2. Use a spoon to scoop out the seeds (save them to snack on!). Drizzle ½ tablespoon of olive oil over the flesh of the squash, along with the pepper and 1 teaspoon of sea salt.

3. Drizzle an additional ½ tablespoon of olive oil on a baking sheet to prevent the squash from sticking. Place them in the oven to bake for about 35-40 minutes.

4. While the squash is cooking, prepare the bread for stuffing. If you haven't already, dice the bread into cubes and set aside. In a large skillet over medium heat, heat the remaining oil. Add the onion and bell peppers to the skillet and sauté until translucent (about 3-5 minutes). Next, add the diced bread, herbs, and all of the spices **EXCEPT** the sugar. Sauté until the bread browns and the edges crisp slightly on one side (about 3-5 minutes). Turn off the heat and set aside until the squash is almost done and tender.

5. In a small- or medium-sized saucepan over medium heat, bring the water and sugar to a boil. Add the pomegranate or cranberries to the pot and reduce the heat to a low to medium heat. Simmer for 10 minutes; the consistency of the sauce (syrupy or not) will depend on which fruit you use. For example, fresh fruit will give you a somewhat syrupy consistency while dried fruit will not.

6. After about 40 minutes (or until the squash becomes tender), remove the squash from the oven. Scoop out half of the flesh from each side and mix into the skillet with the bread. Mix with a large spoon to make a squash stuffing.

7. Use a large spoon to scoop and fill the halves with the stuffing. Place the stuffed squash in the oven for 5 more minutes to crisp the stuffing. Lastly, drizzle the pomegranate (or cranberry) sauce over it, and enjoy.

Cajun Pulled Artichoke 'Chicken' with Dirty Rice

Makes: 2 servings

Ingredients

1 bag of frozen artichoke hearts (12 oz.) (these should be defrosted before use)
3 sprigs of thyme
2 teaspoon of Cajun seasoning
½ teaspoon of paprika
1 teaspoon of garlic powder
1 teaspoon of cayenne pepper
¼ teaspoon of salt and pepper blend

Ingredients for Dirty Rice:

¼ cup each of green bell pepper, celery, & onion (the holy trinity)
1 tablespoon minced garlic
1 minced jalapeño
1 teaspoon of chili powder
2 cups of cooked rice (or you can use a previously frozen bag, or quick cook)
1-2 tablespoon(s) of olive oil
1 teaspoon of oregano (optional)

Directions

1. Add 1-2 tablespoons of olive oil to a large skillet and brown the bell pepper, celery, and onion over medium heat. Once they start to brown and the onions become translucent (about 3-5 minutes), add the rice, garlic, jalapeño, and chili powder. Stir until fully heated throughout, and set aside.

2. Heat a well-oiled cast iron skillet on medium heat for 5-7 minutes.

3. In a large bowl, add the artichoke hearts, seasonings (Cajun seasoning, paprika, garlic powder, cayenne, salt, and pepper) and 2 tablespoons of olive oil and mix them together slightly, while separating or pulling apart the hearts. This will work best if you use your hands!

4. Add the coated artichoke into the cast iron, and press down with a spatula to get a nice, dark sear. Turn it over and brown the other side (about 2 ½ minutes on each side).

5. Remove the artichoke "chicken" from the cast iron pan and serve it over the rice. If you have some on hand, top the dish with parsley as a garnish.

Jerk Cauliflower Chicken Wings

This dish is inspired by the Jamaican jerk blend. It's a mix of Flatbush Brooklyn with a Southern country twang!

Makes: 3 to 4 servings

Ingredients
1 head of cauliflower broken into large florets
¼ cup almond milk + 1 tablespoon of apple cider vinegar
1-2 cups of flour
2 tablespoons of olive oil
2 cups of vegetable oil for frying

Ingredients for Jerk Rub:

2 ½ teaspoons of thyme
2 teaspoons of onion powder
2 teaspoons of black pepper
½ teaspoon of ground cinnamon
½ teaspoon of cayenne pepper
1 teaspoon of salt

Directions

1. In a large bowl, mix all the jerk rub ingredients together with a whisk and set aside.

2. Drizzle the olive oil over the cauliflower florets. Place the florets in the bowl of jerk rub and toss them around to fully coat them.

3. In a large pot or fryer, heat the vegetable oil until it reaches 375°F.

4. Place the flour and 1 tablespoon of the jerk rub into a plastic bag. Gently dunk the cauliflower in the bag of flour. Then dip them in the bowl of milk. Dip them again in the bag and shake the bag to fully coat. Repeat with all the florets. If the flour gets too wet, then add another half cup of flour and more jerk seasoning.

5. Once the oil has reached a temperature of 375°F to 400°F (about 3-5 minutes), drop in the florets and fry for 2-3 minutes, until golden brown on all sides.

6. Remove and drain on a plate lined with a paper towel.

7. Once cool, eat immediately.

Jumpstart Week Two

Now it's your turn! Don't worry, I will start you off…

The key to successful plant-based eating is *to find your own rhythm* that will fit with your accessibility and schedule while ensuring that you eat a varied diet, with nutritious foods that will keep you satisfied. Remember to incorporate a *high-protein source* (such as tofu, seitan, beans, lentils, or chickpeas) into your meals.

While I've included some of my easy-to-follow recipes, you'll notice that some of the meals will be much simpler and don't require you to spend too much time on them, especially during the work-week hustle. You can create your menu from these recipes or mix it them up with veganized versions of your favorite dishes.

The following are ideas for meals and snacks that you can use to plan your meals for a day, or even a full week! This will be very individualized, since you may have requirements that do not allow you to eat certain things due to illness or medication. Check with your doctor or dietician before implementing major dietary changes if you are on a specific diet already.

Here we go!

Weekday Breakfasts

- Toasted English muffins with nut butter (i.e. peanut, almond) and fruit
- Grain vegan bagels with vegan cream cheese, tomatoes, and capers
- **Sweet Potato Toast with Smoky Apple Nut Butter** or other toast with avocado
- Warm cereal bowl, such as oatmeal or cream of wheat
- Smoothie

Weekend Breakfasts

- **Buttermylk Biscuits** and gravy
- Fruit-topped vegan **Pumpkin Pancakes**
- Tofu scramble

Morning Snacks

- Soy or coconut yogurt with nuts or granola
- Mixed fruit bowls, or just single fruits on their own

Weekend Lunches

- Vegan Deli "Meat" pressed, panini-style sandwich
- Chickpea Tuna or **Naw Egg Salad,** in lettuce cups or as a sandwich

- Roasted vegetable grain bowls
- Tacos

Afternoon Snacks

- Handful of nuts
- **Rainbow Carrot Chips**
- Sliced vegetables and hummus or bean dips
- Popcorn with or without vegan butter and your favorite seasoning blend

Weekday Dinners

- Stuffed or grilled portabella mushroom caps
- **Fajita Quesadilla** with peppers, onions, and mushrooms
- Creamy alfredo pasta with spinach or arugula
- Portabella Steak with mashed potatoes
- **Cauliflower Fried "Chicknun"** with collard greens

Weekend Dinners

- Tempeh fried steak
- Popcorn tofu nuggets with potato wedges
- Baked macaroni
- Homemade pizza

Sample Grocery List If You Choose to Follow the Above Suggestions:

1 pack of English Muffins
1 jar of nut butter (such as peanut)
4-5 sweet potatoes/yams
1-2 avocados
3 tomatoes
1 tub of vegan cream cheese
1 pack of tortillas
1-2 pints of soy or coconut yogurt
2-4 different types of fruit to chop and make your own fruit bowls (ex: strawberries, bananas, grapes, apples, cantaloupe)
1 can of pumpkin puree
1 jar of apple jam (or your favorite jam)
1 pack of all-purpose flour
2-3 packs of firm tofu
1 pack of your favorite nuts or nut blend
2 onions
2-3 cans of a variety of beans such as chickpea, black beans etc.

2-3 firm vegetables, such as butternut squash, acorn, and zucchini
1 package of a grain such as rice, farro, quinoa (I know technical quinoa is a seed)
1 lemon
1 pack popcorn kernels
1 vegan chocolate bar
1-2 packs of pasta
6 large portabella mushroom caps
2-3 bunches of greens such as collards, spinach, arugula, kale
1 cauliflower head or florets
2-3 bell peppers
1 bottle of liquid smoke

So, what will week two of plant-based eating look like for you?

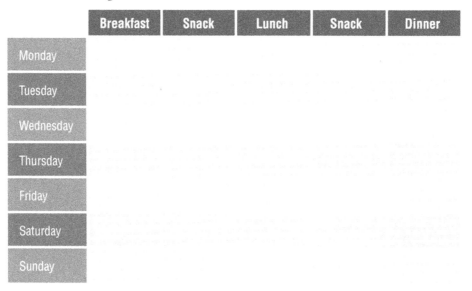

Jumpstart Week Two Meals

	Breakfast	Snack	Lunch	Snack	Dinner
Monday					
Tuesday					
Wednesday					
Thursday					
Friday					
Saturday					
Sunday					

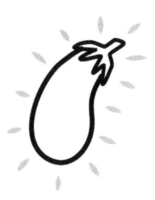

CHAPTER EIGHT

MORE RECIPES: SOUTHERN VEGANS BE GRUBBIN'

It's about to get *real* in your kitchen— Southern-style, y'all!

Snacks

- *Rainbow Carrot Chips*
- *Berbere Dinosaur Kale Chips*
- *Crispy Crunchy Chickpea Snacks*
- *Strawberry Limeade & Mint Bruschetta*
- *Deviled Cremini Mushroom Caps*

Rainbow Carrot Chips

Makes: 4 to 6 servings

Ingredients

1 bag of whole carrots*
1 ½ teaspoons of sea salt
1 teaspoon of pepper
2 tablespoons of olive oil

*If you can find them, try this recipe with rainbow carrots! They are super fun, and kids like to eat colorful food! I encourage using 2 bags because they are so good and go fast!

Directions

1. Preheat oven to 350°F.

2. Wash the carrots thoroughly and slice them lengthwise into long, really thin strips with a mandolin or vegetable peeler.

3. Place the carrot strips in a large bowl and add the salt, pepper, and olive oil. Toss and coat thoroughly.

4. Place the strips on a baking sheet that is lined with parchment paper (if you don't have parchment paper, then you can place them directly on the oven sheet lined with 1 tablespoon of oil or oiled with cooking spray).

5. Bake until the carrots are dry and crispy. Depending on your oven and how thin you sliced them, this can take 25 to 50 minutes. **Start checking them after 25 minutes** to make sure they don't burn. If the edges haven't started to brown after 25 minutes, check them every 10 minutes or so.

6. Let the carrot chips cool for about 5 minutes once they have dried. They will get crisper as they dry. Enjoy!

The above steps are a basic recipe, and you can try playing with different spices and seasonings to suit your cravings. Here are few ideas: berbere Ethiopian seasoning, taco seasoning, or even nutritional yeast for a tangy, cheesy flavor. Use 1-2 teaspoons.

Berbere Dinosaur Kale Chips

Makes: 3 to 4 servings

Ingredients

1 bag of dinosaur kale (although any kale will do)
1 tablespoon of berbere* seasoning. If you can't find this spice, use a Cajun seasoning blend, curry, or jerk seasoning salt.
2 tablespoons of olive oil
½ to 1 teaspoon of salt

*Berbere is an Ethiopian blend made of chili pepper, garlic, fenugreek, rue, and korarima.

Directions

1. Clean the kale leaves by dipping them in cold water and shaking them dry (or use a salad spinner, if you have one). De-stem the kale leaves.

2. Pre-heat the oven to 300°F.

3. Place the kale in a large bowl, along with the remaining ingredients, and toss until they are fully coated and seasoned.

4. Place the chips on a baking sheet carefully, not letting them overlap. Bake for 20-35 minutes, until the chips are crispy and no longer wet.

Crispy Crunchy Chickpea Snacks

Makes: 2 to 4 servings

Ingredients

1 can of cooked garbanzo beans/chickpeas (drained)
3 tablespoons of olive oil
1 teaspoon of lemon juice or apple cider vinegar
2 tablespoons of your favorite seasoning blend that has salt in it (for example, taco seasoning, old bay, or jerk seasoning)

Directions

1. Preheat your oven to 500°F.

2. Drain the can of chickpeas and set it aside. In a large bowl, whisk together 1 tablespoon of the seasoning, all of the vinegar, and all of the olive oil. Drop the chickpeas into the bowl, on top of the marinade. Sprinkle the remaining seasoning on top of the chickpeas.

3. Use a large spoon and toss the chickpeas in the marinade, making sure to fully coat all of the beans.

4. **Drop your oven's temperature down to 300°F***. Spread the seasoned chickpeas on a baking sheet (lined with parchment paper, if you have it). Bake the chickpeas in the oven until they are crispy and have dried out. Depending on your oven and how wet the chickpeas were initially, this can take anywhere from 40-70 minutes. **Check them every 30 minutes.**

5. Store in an airtight container or sandwich bag for a quick on-the-go snack, or use them as a high-protein crouton alternative for salads.

*You want to let it get up to 500°F and then down to 300°F because to ensure you get the best crunchy texture. The high heat will completely dry out the chickpeas, which will be coated in marinade. Lowering the temperature when you put them in will ensure that the get a quick dry and then cook to a crunch at the lower temperature.

Strawberry Limeade & Mint Bruschetta

Makes 4 to 6 servings

Ingredients

1 whole-grain baguette
1 cup fresh minced strawberry
¼ cup of lime juice
1 tablespoon of agave sweetener
2 tablespoons of olive oil
½ teaspoon of salt
1 tablespoon of minced mint

Directions

1. Slice the baguette in thin pieces on a bias (angle).

2. Heat the olive oil in a large skillet and toast the bread pieces. Set aside.

3. In a large bowl, mix all of the remaining ingredients with a fork.

4. Place the mixture on the toast slices and garnish them with the mint.

Deviled Cremini Mushroom Caps

In my pre-vegan days, you wouldn't find me reaching for sweets, chips, ice cream, or candy; instead, I went for the *eggs!* At one point, I was eating SIX eggs a day— and I'm talking about meals with *multiple* types of egg, like an egg white omelet for breakfast with a side of hard-boiled eggs. It was the reason it took me 12 years of being vegetarian to finally make that plunge into veganism.

Needless to say, I'm always looking for ways to vegan-up some type of egg dish. Hence this riff on the deviled egg, all equipped and ready to join you on your next church picnic, family reunion, or baby shower. You can even sneak it into the movies!

Makes: 3 to 4 servings

Ingredients

6-8 cremini mushroom caps (think button mushrooms), cleaned, with the stems and
   gills removed*
1 medium-sized potato (peeled, cut into small dice, and boiled until very soft)
2 tablespoons of mustard
¼ cup of **Basic Vegan Aioli (Mayo)** (See Page 41), or store-bout vegan mayo
1 teaspoon of smoked paprika
¼ teaspoon of ground turmeric
1 teaspoon of sea salt
½ teaspoon of pepper
1 teaspoon of white distilled vinegar (or whatever light vinegar you have in the pantry—
   pretty much anything but balsamic)
1 finely-chopped green onion, for garnish
2 tablespoons of olive oil

*The easiest way to remove the gills is to scoop them out with a small spoon

Directions

1. Preheat the oven to 375°F.

2. Drizzle the olive oil over the cleaned mushroom caps. Sprinkle a pinch of salt on them and bake on a baking sheet in the oven for 7-10 minutes, until they are juicy and starting to release water.

3. While the mushroom caps are baking, make the deviled filling. Place the boiled potato pieces into a large bowl and mash with a spud masher or the back of a heavy ladle. If they are giving you a hard time, add ¼ cup of water or nondairy milk.

4. Whisk the potatoes with a wire whisk or large fork until they are smooth and velvety.

5. Add all of the remaining ingredients **except** the green onions, and whip it good (I couldn't resist that one)! Make sure the whole mixture is yellow and tangy.

6. Using a piping bag or cake-decorating syringe (if you wanna be all fancy, but a small spoon works as well), fill the mushroom caps with the mixture.

7. Top the mushrooms with the chopped chive and an additional dash of paprika.

Sides

- *Loaded Sweet Potato Salad*
- *Church Picnic Broccoli & Apple Coleslaw*
- *Maple Charred Brussel Sprouts with Tempeh Bacon*
- *Italian Pasta Salad*
- *Cauliflower Rice Tabouli Italiano*

Loaded Sweet Potato Salad

Makes: 4 to 8 servings

Ingredients

3-4 medium-to-large sweet potatoes, peeled and medium-diced (about the size of a game dice)
½ to 1 cup of **Basic Vegan Aioli (Mayo)** (See Page 41) (or store-bought vegan mayo) whisked together with ⅓ cup of mustard
¼ cup of diced red onion
¼ cup of diced bell pepper
1 teaspoon thyme
1 minced jalapeño
1-2 teaspoon(s) of salt
½ teaspoon of pepper
½ teaspoon of paprika
2 tablespoons of chopped green onion, for garnish
2 tablespoons of tempeh bacon (optional but highly recommended)

Directions

1. In a large pot, boil the diced sweet potatoes until they are just slightly tender or "al dente." You want them to still be firm so that they don't fall apart.

2. Set in the fridge or freezer for 15-20 minutes to cool.

3. Put all of the potatoes in a large bowl with all of the remaining ingredients (**except** the garnishes). Fold in the aioli thoroughly with a large spoon or rubber spatula.

4. Top with the garnishes and serve chilled.

Church Picnic Broccoli & Apple Coleslaw

Makes: 4 servings

Ingredients

1 head of broccoli (shaved with a vegetable peeler)
1 green apple (sliced thin or with a peeler)
1 teaspoon of salt
1 teaspoon of pepper
½ teaspoon of garlic powder
1 cup of shaved carrot scraps (leftovers from other dishes or shave 2 carrots with a peeler)
¼ to ½ cup of **Basic Vegan Aioli/ Mayo** (See Page 41) recipe or store-bought vegan mayo (amount used will depend on the desired level of creaminess)

Directions

1. Shave the broccoli head, the green apple, and carrot into a large mixing bowl.

2. Add in all of the spices.

3. Pour in the aioli, starting with ¼ cup, and fold together with a small, rubber spatula or a large spoon.

4. If the slaw is still dry or not at the desired creaminess, add more aioli, ¼ cup at a time.

5. Optional: Garnish with ¼ teaspoon of paprika.

Maple Charred Brussel Sprouts with Tempeh Bacon

Makes: 2 to 4 servings

Ingredients

1 bag of fresh Brussels sprouts
¼ block of tempeh
1-2 tablespoon(s) of maple syrup
2 tablespoons of olive oil
1 teaspoon of salt
1 teaspoon of pepper
3 sprigs of thyme or teaspoon of dried thyme

Ingredients for Bacon Marinade:

1 teaspoon of salt
1 tablespoon of apple cider vinegar
1 tablespoon of nutritional yeast
¼ cup of olive oil
2 teaspoons of nut butter (almond or peanut butter works)
½ teaspoon of smoked paprika

Directions

1. Add all of the ingredients for the marinade in a large bowl and whisk them together.

2. Slice the tempeh into thin, bite-sized strips and add them to bowl. Let them marinade in the bowl while you make the Brussel sprouts.

3. Cut the sprouts in half, making sure to remove the bottom, inedible core if your sprouts have them (sometimes, they are already trimmed for you).

4. Put the sprouts in a large bowl and sprinkle with the salt and pepper.

5. Heat an oiled cast-iron skillet on medium heat for 5-7 minutes, until it's just starting to smoke.

6. Pour the oil, maple syrup and thyme over the sprouts in the bowl and mix or toss.

7. Place the sprouts face-down onto the cast iron, pressing down with a spatula to get a hard sear. Once they are browned, flip them over and brown the other side (about 2-5 minutes on each side should do it). Remove and set outside on a napkin or plate.

8. In the same pan that you cooked the sprouts in, add 2 tablespoons of oil and the tempeh "bacon" bits to fry. They should crisp up quickly.

9. Drain the bits on a napkin, crumble them on top of the sprouts, and serve.

Italian Pasta Salad

Makes: 2 to 4 servings

Ingredients

2 cups of cooked pasta
8 sliced black olives
½ green bell pepper sliced thinly
¼ cup diced tomato
1 tablespoon of distilled vinegar (you can substitute with white wine vinegar)
¼ cup of **Basic Vegan Aioli (Mayo)** (See Page 41), or store-bought vegan mayo
1 tablespoon of olive oil
2 tablespoons minced garlic
1 teaspoon of sea salt
1 teaspoon of pepper
¼ teaspoon of oregano
2 tablespoons of minced fresh basil

Directions

1. In a large mixing bowl, add the pasta, vinegar, and all of the vegetables.

2. Pour in the aioli.

3. Add in all of the spices **except** the basil, and mix well.

4. Once everything is fully mixed, taste it and adjust the taste with salt and pepper, if needed.

5. Garnish with the minced basil.

Cauliflower Rice Tabouli Italiano

Makes: 2 to 4 servings

Ingredients

½ head of cauliflower
3 small tomatoes
1 small cucumber
¼ teaspoon of oregano
1 tablespoon of minced garlic
1 teaspoon of salt & pepper blend
2 tablespoons of olive oil
4 tablespoons of water

Directions

1. Using a grater, shave the cauliflower into thin pieces, resembling rice. You can also chop it finely with a large knife.

2. In a medium skillet over medium heat, heat the olive oil garlic, water, and cauliflower rice and sauté for 3-5 minutes. Cool.

3. In a large bowl, pour in the rice and all of the remaining ingredients. Mix well.

4. Chill in the refrigerator.

Breakfast

What Do Vegans Eat for Breakfast?

One question that new plant-based eaters have when they are transitioning from their previous omnivorous lives is what to eat for breakfast. It can be a little tricky to not get stuck in a rut and have some variety that excites your palette. After all, breakfast is the meal that helps you kickstart your day! That being said, the following recipes feature a variety of breakfasts, from savory to sweet and everything in between:

- *Savory Scram*
- *HuevNos Ranchero Toast*
- *Greens, EggZ A' La Cam Toast*
- *Maple Nut Butter & Glazed Peach Toast*
- *Farmer's Skillet Hash*
- *Cream of Barley*
- *Country Breakfast Tofu Ham & Cream of Barley*
- *Buttermylk Biscuits and Black Pepper Mushroom Gravy*
- *Mickey D's Style Tempeh Sausage Biscuit Sandwich with Plum Jam*
- *Berry Blast Smoothie*
- *Breakfast Tostada with Smoky Mango Salsa*
- *Breakfast Burrito Wheels*
- *Sweet Banana Pockets*
- *Peary Dice Oat Bowl*
- *Pumpkin Pancakes*
- *Shredded Savory Skillet Hash Browns*

I dare you to get bored. Go ahead; I'll wait...

Savory Scram

Makes: 2 to 4 servings

Ingredients

1 block of firm tofu (pressed)
1 cup of fresh sliced mushrooms
1 tablespoon of arrowroot or cornstarch
1 teaspoon of garlic powder
2 teaspoons of salt (or 1 tsp of sea salt + 1 tsp of black salt)
½ teaspoon of black pepper
¼ cup of diced onions
2 teaspoons of turmeric powder
4-6 tablespoons of warm water
1 teaspoon of cumin

Directions

1. Slice the tofu block in half, lengthwise, and wrap the pieces in a paper towel. Place the wrapped tofu on a large plate. Set a heavy book or pan on the tofu to press out excess liquid. Set aside.

2. In a small- or medium-sized bowl, whisk together the arrowroot/cornstarch, garlic powder, salt, pepper, turmeric, and, last, the warm water. Set aside.

3. Lay sliced mushrooms on a cutting board and sprinkle with cumin.

4. In a skillet on medium heat, heat the olive oil and add the onions. Sauté the onions until they are translucent, but be careful not to burn them (about 3-5 minutes). Next, add the mushrooms to the skillet and sauté for about 2 minutes.

5. Crumble the tofu and add it to the skillet. Use a slotted spoon to stir and mix the ingredients together.

6. Pour the turmeric mixture into the skillet and stir it into the tofu and vegetable mix.

7. Cook for about 3-5 minutes, until the liquid has cooked off and it resembles scrambled eggs.

8. Serve immediately.

HuevNos Ranchero Toast

Makes: 2 to 4 servings

Ingredients

2 cups of **Savory Scram** (See Page 113)
2-4 slices of your favorite bread toasted (mine is pumpernickel!)
1 cup of fresh, diced tomatoes
½ cup of diced onion
1 diced jalapeño (if spicy ain't your thang, dice ¼ cup of green bell pepper)
¼ cup of minced cilantro or ½ teaspoon of coriander powder
2 tablespoons of olive oil (you can also use cooking spray)
½ sliced avocado for garnish (optional)
Salt to taste

Directions

1. Chop the tomatoes, onion, and jalapeño/pepper into a small dice and mix together in a small bowl. Add the cilantro/coriander and a pinch of salt to the bowl and stir. Set pico de gallo aside.

2. Heat 1 tablespoon of olive oil (or cooking spray) in a large skillet on medium heat. Add the **Savory Scram** to the skillet, and warm until fully cooked.

3. Toast the bread in a toaster or brown in a skillet with one tablespoon of olive oil or cooking spray.

4. To assemble, lay toast on a cutting board. Use a large spoon and add the scram evenly onto each slice. Next, top each piece with the pico de gallo. Garnish with the avocado slices, if using.

Greens, EggZ A' La Cam Toast

When I was a kid, my favorite book (besides *The Three Billy-Goats Gruff*) was *Green Eggs & Ham*. For some reason, the thought of eating green eggs was appealing to my 6-year-old self. Although I'll never eat them in a car, or on a bar, or under the stars, this veganized version will definitely satisfy an egg craving!

Makes: 2 to 4 servings

Ingredients

2 cups of **Savory Scram** (See Page 113)
2 cups of fresh chopped kale, or your favorite green
2-4 slices of your favorite bread, toasted
2 teaspoons of garlic powder or 1 tablespoon of fresh minced garlic
2 tablespoons of olive oil
1 teaspoon of sea salt
½ teaspoons of black pepper
1 teaspoon of dried parsley flakes (you can substitute this with fresh, minced parsley
  or dried thyme if you prefer)
1 squeezed lemon wedge and its zest (optional to garnish greens; it gives a
  nice citrus pop)
 ½ sliced avocado, for garnish (optional)

Directions

1. Place the greens in a large bowl and add the garlic powder, salt, and pepper.

2. In a large skillet on medium heat, heat one tablespoon of olive oil. Add the greens to the skillet and lightly sauté using tongs (or a slotted spoon) to stir. Sauté for 2-3 minutes. You want the greens to wilt, but not get mushy. Remove them from the skillet and set aside. If using, garnish with the lemon juice and zest from the lemon wedge.

3. Place an additional tablespoon of olive oil into the skillet (on medium heat) and add the **Savory Scram.** Use a slotted spoon and stir the scram to heat it evenly throughout. Heat until fully cooked.

4. Toast the bread in a toaster or brown in an oiled skillet.

5. To assemble, lay the toast flat on a cutting board. Next, lay the greens on top of the toast, distributing them evenly among all slices. Scoop the scram evenly onto each piece.

6. If using, top with the sliced avocado. Sprinkle additional salt and pepper to taste, and add the parsley flakes.

Maple Nut Butter & Glazed Peach Toast

Makes: 2 to 4 servings

Ingredients

2-4 slices of your favorite bread, toasted
2 firm peaches
½ cup of nut butter (such as peanut butter or almond butter)
2 tablespoons of maple syrup
½ teaspoon of vanilla extract
2 tablespoons of non-dairy vegan butter
2 teaspoons of brown sugar
1 teaspoon of cinnamon

Directions

1. Remove the pit from the peaches and slice into ¼-inch-thick slices.

2. In a bowl, whisk the maple syrup and vanilla extract with the nut butter together. Set aside.

3. In a sauté pan, on medium heat, melt the vegan butter. Once melted, add the brown sugar and cinnamon. Whisk it all to mix well.

4. Add the peaches to the sauté pan and coat them in the glaze using a large spoon or rubber spatula. Cook for 2-3 minutes until the peaches get slightly tender, but not mushy. Remove them from the pan.

5. Toast the bread using a toaster, or add a tablespoon of vegan butter to a skillet and brown the bread on it for a couple of minutes on each side.

6. To assemble, spread the maple butter onto each slice of toasted bread and then top with the glazed peaches.

Farmer's Skillet Hash

This rustic, homey dish is so versatile that you can have it for breakfast and dinner (or as I like to call it, brinner!). All you gotta do is scoop a heaping spoonful into a warm tortilla toasted on an open flame (Is there any other way to toast a tortilla?). Top it with some hot sauce and fresh cilantro, and damn! It's super easy and delicious dish to treat yourself or someone else to a homey vegan meal.

Makes: 3 to 4 servings

Ingredients

4-6 medium-to-large potatoes, diced to a small or medium size
2 medium-to-large sweet potatoes, diced in a similar shape
½ a red onion, diced in a similar size to the potatoes
1 diced jalapeno
1 cup of **Meaty Lone Star Tempeh Chili** (See Page 143) (optional, but it tastes banging in this dish!)
½ cup of diced tomato
2 sprigs of fresh thyme
1 ½ teaspoons of sea salt
1 teaspoon of paprika
1 teaspoon of ground sage
2 tablespoons of olive oil
2 tablespoons of chopped, fresh cilantro, for garnish

Directions

1. Preheat the oven to 375°F, and place a well-seasoned skillet in the oven.

2. Place the potatoes and all of the other items EXCEPT the cilantro and the chili (if using) in a large bowl.

3. Mix well with a large spoon until all of the potatoes and vegetables are fully coated with the spices and olive oil (We don't want no ashy potatoes!).

4. **Make sure to use a thick pot holder when handling the cast iron; it will be _extremely_ hot!** Remove the skillet from the oven. Pour the hash in the heated skillet and roast for 25 to 30 minutes. Once the hash is almost fully cooked and the onions are browning, add the chili to the top of the hash and heat in the oven for an additional 5-10 minutes.

5. Remove the skillet from the oven. Try one of the potatoes to make sure they are fully cooked.

6. Garnish with the cilantro and serve it in a bowl with some hot sauce or in a tortilla.

Cream of Barley

This comfort-in-a-bowl is modeled after Cream of Wheat.

Makes: 1 serving

Ingredients

1 cup of cooked barley (if using from a previously frozen batch), or use quick cook barley and follow package instructions (you can also use another grain such as farro, rice, or polenta)
½ cup of nondairy milk (try a fortified one for a B12 boost)
½ cup of **Basic Cashew Cream** (See Page 42)
½ teaspoon of cinnamon
2 tablespoons of dried fruit (such as cranberries or raisins)
1 tablespoon chopped nuts, for garnish (optional)

Directions

1. In a medium saucepan over medium heat, heat the cooked barley in the non-dairy milk for about 3 minutes.

2. Stir in the cashew cream and reduce the heat to low, stirring constantly for a rich and creamy texture. Cook for an additional 5 to 7 minutes.

3. Add the cinnamon. Garnish with the dried fruit and nuts.

Country Breakfast Tofu Ham & Cream of Barley

When I was a kid, the main breakfast staple we had was rice (with sugar in it, of course) and wieners. Talk about a country breakfast! It was cheap, quick and easy. This version uses a more sophisticated grain— barley— topped with tofu ham instead.

Makes: 2 servings

Ingredients

½ block of extra-firm tofu (sliced into 4-5 steaks, about ½ an inch thick each)
¼ cup of beet juice
1 cup of **Cream of Barley** (See Page 120)

Ingredients for the Ham Marinade:

½ cup of olive oil
2 tablespoons of nut butter (I used almond butter)
½ teaspoon of molasses (optional)
1 tablespoon of salt
1 tablespoon apple cider vinegar
1 teaspoon of garlic powder

Directions

1. Place all of the marinade ingredients in a large bowl and whisk together. Set aside.

2. Pour the beet juice in a small bowl. Dip the tofu steaks into the beet juice to stain. Then, place tofu in the large bowl and completely coat with the marinade. Let stand for 10 minutes.

3. Heat a well-oiled cast iron on medium heat for 8 minutes.

4. Place the marinated tofu on the cast-iron pan, pressing down firmly with a spatula. Once it starts to get a dark color and sear (about 4-5 minutes), flip over and repeat.

5. Once both sides are fully cooked, set aside to cool on a plate.

6. Enjoy with the **Cream of Barley** from the previous recipe.

Buttermylk Biscuits and Black Pepper Mushroom Gravy

Ain't nothing more Southern Comfort than a moist, fluffy buttermilk biscuit. While growing up, I remember watching my mom pop open one of those biscuit dough tubes and baking them on a cookie sheet. I thought that was the business, straight-up! However, out of the necessity of having to make more of my own things from scratch, I created my own go-to recipe. There's nothing like customizing a biscuit mix and adding any flavors you want! Once you make biscuits from scratch, you'll never go back.

Makes: 6 to 8 biscuits

Ingredients

Ingredients for Biscuits:

2 cups of all-purpose flour
¾ cup of non-dairy milk mixed with 1 tablespoon of apple cider vinegar
1 tablespoon of baking powder
½ teaspoon of baking soda
1 teaspoon of salt
¼ cup of vegan butter

Ingredients for Black-Pepper Mushroom Gravy:

1 cup of flour
¼ cup of olive oil (can sub with mild-flavored vegetable oil) + 1 tablespoon of olive oil
2 teaspoons of black pepper
1 teaspoon of salt
1 teaspoon of garlic powder
½ cup of diced onion
½ cup of chopped mushroom scraps (or gills left over from other dishes)
½ to 1 cup of vegetable stock

Directions

For Biscuits

1. Preheat oven to 450°F. In a small bowl, curdle the non-dairy milk with a tablespoon of apple cider vinegar (this will make the "buttermilk").

2. In a large bowl, mix all of the dry ingredients together with a whisk or a large fork. Crumble the cold butter into the bowl until it gets pebbly.

3. Make a well in the center of the mixture and pour in the wet ingredients. Using a spoon, mix well, until the texture goes from a wet batter to a moist dough.

4. On a lightly-floured surface, place a dough ball in the center and knead it for about 5 minutes.

5. Slightly roll out the dough to flatten. Using a cookie cutter (or my preferred method, the top of a glass), cut out circles of dough and place the biscuit pieces on a lightly-oiled baking sheet.

6. Bake for 12 to 15 minutes, until they are fluffy and golden brown.

For Gravy

1. In a large skillet over medium heat, sauté the mushroom scraps and onions until they have browned (about 2-3 minutes).

2. Pour in the flour and *slowly* pour in the olive oil. As it starts to clump and form a "roux," turn down the heat slightly.

3. Whisk in the vegetable stock, ¼ of a cup at a time, while constantly whisking to thin out the roux.

4. Continue to pour in more stock until you reach the desired consistency of your gravy. Personally, I prefer a thinner, more uniform gravy that isn't very lumpy.

5. Add the salt, pepper, and garlic powder to seasoning.

6. Turn down the heat to low and let it keep heating until you are ready to serve.

Mickey D's Style Tempeh Sausage Biscuit Sandwich with Plum Jam

When I was in elementary school, when a certain bus driver used to take us through the McDonald's drive-thru (not really sure of the legality of that, since we shoulda been on our way to school!), my favorite thing to get was the sausage biscuit sandwich with grape jelly. Even as a child, I knew the flavor combination of savory, silky, and sweet was the way to go. Although I am lucky enough to be able to choose not to partake in the heavily-processed world that is fast food anymore, this vegan riff definitely brings back some sweet food memories.

Makes: 2 sandwiches

Ingredients

Ingredients for Sandwich:

1-2 homemade **Buttermylk Biscuits** (See Page 122)
2 tempeh squares or fillets
2 teaspoons of cumin
1 tablespoon of finely-minced fennel seed (can sub for ½ teaspoon of ground fennel)
1 teaspoon of sage
1 teaspoon of maple syrup
1 teaspoon of pepper
2 teaspoons of salt
¼ cup of mild vegetable oil

Ingredients for Jam: (optional, as you can use store-bought)

1 cup of fresh, chopped plum
½ cup of water
1 teaspoon of agave syrup

Directions

For Jam (if making your own)

1. Combine all of the ingredients in a medium saucepan and bring to a boil.

2. Once it starts to boil, reduce the temperate to low and simmer until most of the liquid has evaporated.

3. Stir the jam. Once it reaches a jam consistency, remove from heat.

4. Store in a jar in the fridge for about 2 weeks.

For Tempeh Sausage

1. Heat the oil in a small pan on low heat for 2-3 minutes (if the oil is popping, then it's too hot!). Turn off the heat.

2. In a large bowl, whisk all of the spices together.

3. Dip the tempeh fillets in the warm oil. Then, place them in the bowl of spices and completely coat them with the "sausage" rub.

4. In a large skillet, heat 1 tablespoon of olive oil on medium heat. Place the tempeh in the skillet and press down with a spatula to brown.

5. Once it's golden brown, flip it over and repeat on the other side (about X minutes per side).

6. Slice the biscuits in half and reheat in the oven for 3-5 minutes at 300°F.

7. Smear on the jam, add the tempeh, and enjoy!

Berry Blast Smoothie

Makes: 1 to 2 smoothies

Ingredients

1 banana
1 cup of orange juice
1 cup of cold water
1 cup of frozen or fresh berries (this can be a berry blend or all one type, such as strawberries)
½ cup of spinach (optional)
1 cup of ice, if you are not using frozen berries

Directions

1. Pour the water and orange juice into the blender.

2. Add the banana, berries, spinach, and ice, if using.

3. Turn the blender to a low speed and blend for a few seconds.

4. Incrementally increase the speed and blend until you reach the desired smoothness and texture.

5. Serve immediately.

Breakfast Tostada with Smoky Mango Salsa

Makes: 2 to 4 servings

Ingredients

4 corn tortillas
2 cups of **Savory Scram** (See Page 113)
1 can of cooked refried beans
1 cup of shredded lettuce, such as iceberg (any green will work)
2 tablespoons of vegetable oil

Ingredients for Mango Salsa:

1 fresh mango
½ cup of diced red onion
1 teaspoon of smoked paprika
1 teaspoon of liquid smoke
1 small, fresh, diced tomato
1 diced jalapeno
1 teaspoon of sea salt

Directions

1. Preheat the oven to 375°F.

2. For salsa, peel the skin off of the mango with a veggie peeler. Cut the flesh off of the large, flat pit and dice the flesh.

3. In a medium-sized bowl, add the mango, diced onion, diced jalapeño, diced tomato, smoked paprika, liquid smoke, and salt. Mix with a large spoon and set aside.

For Tostadas

1. Lay tortillas flat on a baking sheet and drizzle 1 tablespoon of oil over all of the tortillas. Put the sheet into the preheated oven. Bake for 5-7 minutes (check them after 5 minutes, since ovens vary), flip, and repeat on the other side. They should be golden and crisp. Once they have reached this point, turn the oven off, but leave them in to stay warm and crisp longer.

2. Cook the beans in a medium saucepan.

3. In a large skillet over medium heat, heat 1 tablespoon of olive oil. Heat the scram in the oil for 3-5 minutes, until it is fully warmed throughout.

4. To assemble, remove the tortilla shells from the oven. Smear a generous amount of beans onto each shell. Next, top the beans with the shredded lettuce. Evenly distribute the scram on top of the beans and shredded lettuce.

5. Top with the mango salsa.

Breakfast Burrito Wheels

Makes: 2 to 4 servings

Ingredients

1 can of cooked black beans (you can substitute with your choice of cooked
    bean)
1-2 large tortillas or wraps
2 cups of **Savory Scram** (See Page 113)
2 cups of fresh spinach (or fresh chopped kale)
½ cup of diced tomatoes
¼ cup of diced onion
1 diced jalapeño pepper
1 tablespoon of olive oil

Directions

1. In a medium saucepan, cook the beans.

2. In a large skillet on medium heat, heat the olive oil. Add the scram to warm
    it up (about 3-5 minutes).

3. Heat the tortillas by placing them directly onto the stovetop burner. Char for
    about 20   to 30 seconds on each side.

4. Remove from the flame. Place the spinach onto the tortilla. Then add the
    beans,
    the scram, and top them with the fresh, diced veggies.

5. Roll the burrito up tightly, starting on one side and rolling it into itself, cigar-
    style.

6. Cut the burrito into 3-5 one-inch-thick segments.

7. Stand the wheels on a plate and top with hot sauce, your favorite salsa, or try
    my **Smoky Mango Salsa** recipe (See Page 127).

Sweet Banana Pockets

Makes: 2 to 4 servings

Ingredients

2-4 tortillas or wraps
2 sliced bananas
2 tablespoons of non-dairy vegan butter
½ teaspoon of nutmeg
½ teaspoon of cinnamon
¼ to ½ cup of nut butter (such as almond butter)
2-4 tablespoons of jam or preserves
1 tablespoon of cooking oil, plus 1 additional tablespoon of vegan butter or cooking
  spray to prevent sticking
1 tablespoon of powdered sugar, for garnish (optional)

Directions

1. Melt 2 tablespoons of the vegan butter in a saucepan on medium heat (you
    can use a microwave, if you prefer).

2. Transfer the melted butter into a small bowl. Add the bananas, nutmeg, and
    cinnamon to the bowl. Mix with a spoon.

3. Lay a tortilla/wrap flat on a cutting board. Starting lengthwise on 1 half of the
    tortilla, spread some of the maple nut butter. Along the other half of the tortilla,
    spread some of the jam. Place the some of the banana slices on the jam side.

4. Fold the nut butter side on top of the jam side so that it resembles a calzone.
    Press along the edges to seal. Repeat with the remaining ingredients.

5. In a large skillet over medium heat, add 1 tablespoons oil, vegan butter or use
    cooking spray so that the pocket doesn't stick.

6. Place the pocket in the skillet to brown. Press it down with a spatula, and sear
    for 2-3 minutes on each side.

7. Garnish with the powdered sugar if you are using it.

Peary Dice Oat Bowl

Makes: 1 to 2 servings

Ingredients

¼ cup of uncooked oats
¾ cup of water (to cook oats)
1 fresh pear, sliced and cored
2 tablespoons of vegan butter
½ teaspoons of cinnamon
1 tablespoon of brown sugar
1 cup of diced tempeh

Ingredients for Bacony Marinade:

¼ cup of olive oil or vegetable oil
2 teaspoons of sea salt
1 teaspoon of peanut butter
2 teaspoons of apple cider vinegar
1 tablespoon of nutritional yeast
1 teaspoon of molasses (optional)
1 tablespoon of olive oil or cooking spray for frying

Directions

1. In a medium saucepan, cook oats according to directions.

2. In a small- or medium-sized bowl, whisk together all of the marinade ingredients. Add the tempeh to the marinade and mix with a spoon to fully coat the tempeh in the marinade. Set it aside to let it marinate further.

3. In a medium- or large-sized skillet over medium heat, melt the vegan butter. Once melted, whisk in the cinnamon and brown sugar.

4. Add the pear slices to the skillet and cook in the glaze (about 3-5 minutes). The pears should be slightly glossy and tender, but not mushy. Remove from the pan and set aside.

5. In the same skillet, heat the tablespoon of olive oil (or cooking spray). Add the tempeh and cook in the oil until browned and slightly tender (about 5 minutes).

6. Lastly, place the cooked oats in a bowl, and arrange the glazed pear slices along the middle of the oats.

7. Garnish the bowl with the tempeh "bacon" and enjoy!

Pumpkin Pancakes

Makes: 2 to 4 servings

Ingredients

2 cups of flour
1½ cups of non-dairy milk + 1 tablespoon of apple cider vinegar
1 tablespoon of melted vegan butter
2 teaspoons of baking powder
1 teaspoon of baking soda
3 tablespoons of raw or brown sugar
1 teaspoon of salt
1 cup of canned pumpkin (can substituted with 1 cup of cooked, mashed sweet potato)
1 teaspoon of vanilla extract
2 additional tablespoons of vegan butter or cooking spray, to prevent pancakes from sticking

Directions

1. Whisk the non-dairy milk and vinegar together in a small bowl and set aside.

2. Melt 1 tablespoon of vegan butter in a small saucepan.

3. In a large bowl, whisk the flour, salt, baking soda, baking powder, and sugar together

4. In a separate large bowl, whisk the canned pumpkin, vegan butter, non-dairy milk, and vanilla extract together.

5. Using a sifter, fine mesh, or fine strainer, sift the flour into the bowl of wet ingredients.

6. Mix everything into a batter using a large spoon or rubber spatula. If batter is too thick, thin it out with an additional ¼ cup of non-dairy milk.

7. Spray a large skillet with cooking oil, or add 1-2 tablespoons of vegan butter to it and melt the butter over medium heat. Make sure the pan isn't too hot (as in smoking), because you don't want to scorch the outside of the pancakes before the inside is cooked!

8. Use a ladle to scoop out a large spoonful of the batter onto the hot skillet. Once the pancake starts to bubble, using a fast movement and a flat spatula, slide it under the pancake and flip it. Cook on this side for about 2 minutes, pressing it down with the spatula.

9. It should take 2-3 minutes each side to cook. Tear off a little piece on the side of one to taste and check if it's done. **Note:** They will be slightly more moist than regular pancakes because of the pumpkin!

10. Repeat with the remaining batter. Top with my **Maple Butter** recipe (See Page 117), or with your favorite syrup.

Shredded Savory Skillet Hash Browns

Makes: 4 servings

Ingredients

1 bag of frozen, shredded potatoes (if you can't find these, peel 4 large potatoes and shred them on a cheese grater)
½ cup of fresh, diced tomatoes
1 cup of sautéed mushrooms
½ cup of diced onion
½ cup of diced bell peppers
1 teaspoon of cumin
1-2 teaspoons of garlic powder
1-2 teaspoons of sea salt
1 teaspoon of black pepper
2-3 tablespoons of olive oil
1 diced jalapeño (optional, but recommended)

Directions

1. Heat 1 tablespoon of olive oil in a cast iron skillet on medium heat.

2. Preheat your oven's broiler.

3. In a small bowl, whisk cumin, 1 teaspoon of garlic powder, 1 tablespoon of olive oil, and ½ teaspoon of pepper. Add the mushrooms to coat them.

4. In a separate large skillet (not the cast iron), heat 1 tablespoon of olive oil along with the onion, bell peppers, and jalapeño (if using). Sauté using a large slotted spoon for about 3-5 minutes. Onions should be translucent, and the other vegetables should be slightly tender.

5. Add the mushroom to the skillet with the aromatics (onions and peppers) and sauté them until they are tender (about 3-5 minutes).

6. Lay a thin layer of the hash browns onto the cast iron skillet (about half of the bag). Let them brown and stick to the pan without stirring too much (about 3-5 minutes).

7. Place the sautéed veggies on top of the potatoes and place the remaining potatoes on top of the veggies.

8. Drizzle the remaining tablespoon of olive oil on top of the hash browns and sprinkle them with a dash of salt (about ½ to 1 teaspoon).

9. Place the skillet in the broiler for the hash to brown. This should take 6-12 minutes; **check every 3-5 minutes,** since broilers singe foods quite fast. **Note:** Make sure to handle with thick pot holders, because the handle will be   extremely hot!

10. Serve the hash browns with a dollop of my **Basic Cashew Cheese** (See Page 42), and then add the sliced jalapeños, salsa, or good old hot sauce. If you're really country, like me, use ketchup instead!

Lunch and Dinner

Protein Heavyweight Meals

If you are concerned about not getting enough protein due to removing meat from your diet (you really don't have to be!), this next section has you covered. The recipes in this section are high in protein content and even higher on the deliciousness scale:

- *ChickNun Enchiladas*
- *Meaty Lone Star Tempeh Chili*
- *M-Square Frito Pie*
- *Sweet Pea Fritter*
- *Eggplant Pasta Sheet Lasagna Stacks*
- *Homemade Seitan*
- *Homemade Seitan Short Ribs in a Bourbon Barbecue Sauce with Sautéed Collards and Tofu Damn Hock Strips*
- *Pea Butter Pesto*
- *Louisiana-Style Cornmeal-Encrusted Tofu Fish Fry*
- *Fiya Fiya CamBalaya*
- *Sesame Rocking Reuben Sandwich*
- *Smoked Baked Macaroni & Cheese*
- *Tempalo ChickNun Club Salad with Tofu Feta and Vegan Hunty Mustard*

Now, dive in! Who knows, after switching to eating plants, you might just feel strong enough to lift a few trees!

ChickNun Enchiladas

Makes: 3 to 4 servings

Ingredients

6-8 tortillas (small- to medium-sized)
2-3 tablespoons of canola or vegetable oil
1 cup of **Quick, Creamy Cashew Cheese** (See Page 43)
2-3 cups of a fresh green, such as arugula, spinach, or kale
½ cup of diced tomato, for garnish (optional)
1 can of jackfruit in water (artichoke hearts will work, also)

Ingredients for Chicken Marinade:

¼ cup of olive or mild vegetable oil
1 teaspoon of paprika
1 teaspoon of poultry seasoning
1 teaspoon of apple cider vinegar

Ingredients for Enchilada Sauce:

1 can of kidney beans, cooked
2 tablespoons of taco seasoning
1 fresh red pepper
1 teaspoon of coriander powder **or** 2 tablespoons of minced cilantro
½ to 1 cup of water

Directions

For Chicken Marinade

1. Add all of the marinade ingredients **EXCEPT** the jackfruit (or artichoke hearts) into a large bowl and whisk.

2. Drain the can of jackfruit (or artichoke). Chop jackfruit or artichoke until they have a shredded or chopped meat consistency. If using jackfruit, remove the seeds and end pieces completely if they are too firm to mince. Otherwise, you can also chop into chunks if that makes it easier. Add the jackfruit (or artichoke) to the marinade bowl and set aside.

For the Enchilada Sauce

1. Pour the beans into a medium saucepan or pot. Add the taco seasoning and cook the beans.

2. Let the beans cool for 2-3 minutes. Add the beans, red pepper, cilantro/coriander, and water to a blender. Blend for 2-3 minutes, incrementally going from a low to medium speed until you have a slightly thin, creamy sauce. If it is too thick and more like a paste, and ½ cup more of water and blend again. Set aside.

Note: This sauce freezes well, so feel free to make extra!

For Enchiladas

1. Preheat the oven to 375°F.

2. Heat 1 tablespoon of oil in a cast iron skillet over medium heat. Add the jackfruit (or artichoke) to the skillet and let it stick. (Don't stir for the first few minutes, so that it sears and gets a nice, developed, roasted taste.) Fully cook the jackfruit (or artichoke) for about 5-8 minutes. If you aren't sure if it's fully cooked, remove a small piece and taste it. It should be tender and slightly browned from the char.

3. Heat the remaining tablespoons of oil in a large skillet over medium heat (you can use the same skillet if you remove the jackfruit/artichoke first). Place the tortillas in the oil, one at a time, to heat. Just warm them to make them more malleable; do not to fry them (about 1 minute on each side). Remove them with tongs and place them on a plate lined with a paper towel.

4. In a casserole pan, pour a generous amount of the bean sauce on the bottom of the pan (at least ½ cup). Assemble the enchiladas by spreading a spoonful of the **Creamy Cashew Cheese** along the middle of a tortilla. Next, spread a few leaves of the greens along the line of the cashew cheese, followed by a row of the jack ChickNun. Roll the enchilada up, cigar-style.

5. Place the enchilada seam-side-down into the casserole pan. Repeat the process with the remaining ingredients. Line them in a row in the pan. Pour the remaining ½ cup of the sauce along the middle of the enchiladas.

6. Bake for 10 minutes.

7. Garnish with tomatoes and serve immediately.

Note: This recipe freezes well, so make extra and stock up. You can thank me later!

Meaty Lone Star Tempeh Chili

This recipe takes about 30-45 minutes and makes 1.5 quarts. It can be frozen, so make extra for busy days.

Tip: Serve with elbow macaroni for homemade hamburger helper!

Makes: 4 servings

Ingredients

For the Spice Blend:

1 teaspoon of cumin
1 teaspoon of salt
1 teaspoon of pepper
1 teaspoon of chili powder
1 teaspoon of paprika
½ teaspoon of cayenne pepper
¼ teaspoon of cinnamon

For Chili:

1 8-ounce package of tempeh
2 cups of cooked farro
1 cup of vegetable stock
2 ripe tomatoes
1 jalapeño
½ large, red onion
2 minced garlic cloves
2 tablespoons of olive oil

Directions

Optional: Toss the jalapeño, onion, and tomato in 1 tablespoon of olive oil and blister in the broiler for 3-5 minutes for depth of flavor.

1. Start a large pot with 2 cups of water to boil. Once it is boiling, drop the heat to medium and add the farro. Cook the farro until tender according to the package instructions.

2. Crumble the tempeh in a bowl and season it with the spice blend. You can leave some of the pieces bigger (about the size of a quarter) for a meatier texture.
3. In a large skillet over medium heat, add 1 tablespoon of olive oil and sauté the tempeh mixture with the minced garlic until slightly brown (about 3-5 minutes).

4. Place the cooked farro in a pot and add the tempeh, diced vegetables, and stock. Mix well.

5. Cook for about 20 to 30 minutes on medium heat, stirring occasionally, until it is a thick, chili consistency and most of the liquid has evaporated.

6. Taste it, and add 1 to 2 teaspoons of salt and pepper if desired.

M-Square Frito Pie

The very first time I had the Southern Stadium classic Frito Pie, I was at a football game in Marlin, Texas— otherwise known as M-Square. It's normally runny, meaty chili, Fritos corn chips, and onions, served in the bag of chips with a spork! Here's my version, using the slightly sweet crisp from homemade plantain chips. Although I'd like to think my taste has gotten a bit more sophisticated since I was that 9-year-old Texas girl, sometimes you can't take the country out of me!

Makes: 3 to 4 servings

Ingredients

2 cups of the *Meaty Lone Star Tempeh Chili* (See Page 143)
¼ cup of diced red onions (from the left over half from making the chili in the previous recipe)
2 large, green plantains, for chips (fresh ones are usually found in the produce section, but you can use store-bought corn chips instead)
1-2 cups of vegetable oil, for frying
salt to taste

Directions

1. Using a small paring knife, cut along the ridges and edges of the plantain. Slide a butter knife (or your thumb) under the ridges to peel the green skin off of the plantain.

2. Lay the plantain down horizontally on a cutting board and slice (shave) the plantain into long, thin strips with a vegetable peeler. It is easiest if you hold the very tip of the plantain with one hand while shaving it.

3. Heat the oil in a medium-to-large saucepan or fryer until the heat reaches between 375-400°F. If you don't have a thermometer, then, once you start hearing the oil sizzle, throw in one "chip." If floats, then the grease is hot enough.

4. Being careful not to overload the pot, fry the chips, turning them over until they are golden on each side (about 30 secs to 2 minutes per side, depending on the thickness of your chips).

5. Drain the chips on a napkin.

6. Heat the chili in a separate pot on the stove.

7. To assemble, get a bowl or a small basket and fill it with the chips. Add the chili over the chips. Top the whole thing with diced onions. For that true Texas experience, top it all with sliced jalapeños.

Sweet Pea Fritter

Make these fritters, and you'll have everyone saying pass the peas!

Makes: 3 to 4 servings

Ingredients

2-3 cups of frozen peas, cooked
½ cup of diced red onions
1½ cups of breadcrumbs
1 tablespoon of ground flaxseed + 2 tablespoons of warm water (FLEGG, remember?)
2 teaspoons of salt
1 teaspoon of pepper
1 teaspoon of garlic powder
1-2 cups of vegetable oil, for frying

Directions

1. Cook the peas in 1 cup of water or stock on medium heat until tender (about 3-5 minutes).

2. After draining the peas, place them in a large bowl and mash them with a potato masher, or with the back of a heavy ladle or spoon.

3. Add the onions, seasonings, breadcrumbs, and FLEGG to the bowl and mix well with a slotted spoon or large soup spoon.

4. In a medium-to-large saucepan or fryer, heat the vegetable oil until it reaches 375°F. Using an ice-cream scooper or spoon, scoop the mixture into the hot grease. Fry for about 2 minutes on each side, or until all sides are golden brown.

5. Drain on a napkin.

Eggplant Pasta Sheet Lasagna Stacks

I have so many fond memories of my mom opening the big-ass block of Stouffer's and popping it in the oven. I also remember that if I had forgotten to take it out of the freezer before she got home, it would be, like, 17 hours before we ate because it took so ridiculously long to cook! I created this version using thinly-sliced eggplant instead of pasta sheets to add more flavor, volumize the dish, and save on the simple carbs!

Makes: 2 to 4 servings

Ingredients

1 large, peeled eggplant
1 cup of **Quick, Creamy Cashew Cheese** (See Page 43)
½ cup of sautéed tempeh
1 teaspoon of cumin
½ teaspoon of salt
½ teaspoon of pepper
1 cup of sautéed kale (or desired green; spinach and arugula also work)
2 garlic cloves, chopped
3 tablespoons of olive oil

Ingredients for Marinara Sauce:

2 ripe fresh tomatoes
1 cup of sundried tomatoes
¼ cup of diced onions
¼ to ½ cup of vegetable stock
¼ cup of minced basil
1 teaspoon of salt
1 teaspoon of pepper
¼ cup of cooking wine; red or white table wine also works (optional, but adds amazing depth of flavor)

Directions

For Marinara Sauce

1. Dice the tomato into large chunks and lightly season them with salt and pepper.

2. Pour 1 tablespoon of olive oil into a large saucepan. Add the tomato and onion. Brown them for 2-3 minutes.

3. Just as the tomato is starting to stick, *deglaze* (loosen the tomato from sticking) by pouring in the cooking wine and cooking down for 3-5 minutes.

4. Add the stock, basil, and sundried tomatoes and cook down until half of the liquid has evaporated.

5. Remove the pot from the heat, and let it cool for about 5 minutes.

6. Put the sauce in a blender and pulse it on a low speed until it reaches a chunky consistency. If you prefer a thinner sauce, pulse it for longer.

For Lasagna

1. Preheat the oven to 400°F.

2. Slice the eggplant lengthwise into long strips resembling lasagna noodles.

3. Place the lasagna "pasta" in a bowl and toss it with a tablespoon of olive oil and ½ teaspoon of salt and pepper. Set aside.

4. Sauté the kale in a skillet with olive oil and 2 chopped garlic cloves. Remove from heat.

5. Using the same skillet, sauté the tempeh crumbles with the teaspoon of cumin and the other ½ teaspoon of salt and pepper.

To Assemble

1. Lay down one layer of the eggplant sheets in a wide casserole pan. Next, add a layer of sauce and tempeh. Add more sheets and smear with a spoonful of cashew cheese and top with a few leaves of kale.

2. Repeat the process over until you have used all of the ingredients.

3. Top the lasagna with a thin layer of sauce.

4. Bake in the oven for 30 minutes, until the edges have browned and the eggplant is fully cooked.

Homemade Seitan

This is a vegan mainstay. You can make everything from faux turkey loaves for holidays to fried Ficken (fake chicken), faux ribs, faux brisket, and so much more with this stuff! It's packed full of protein and really easy to make. Once you have this basic recipe down, you can tweak it any which way imaginable.

Cook time should be between 50 and 75 minutes. You can make large batches to freeze in airtight containers. To defrost, move the frozen containers to the fridge.

Makes: 4 servings

Ingredients

2 cups of vital wheat gluten*
1 cup of nutritional yeast**
2 teaspoons of sea salt
1 teaspoon of pepper
1 teaspoon of thyme (fresh or dried works)
1 teaspoon of paprika
¼ cup of onion (you can replace with 1 teaspoon of onion or garlic powder)
1 cup of vegetable stock
1 tablespoon of Bragg's Liquid Aminos (you can substitute with soy sauce if you don't
    have Bragg's)
2 tablespoons of olive oil
1 teaspoon of molasses (optional; it is used to rub on the outside of the loaf, for color)

*You can find vital wheat gluten in the baking or flour sections of grocery stores. Vital wheat gluten comes in a flour form (the most popular commercially-available kind is from Bob's Red Mill), and it has a high protein content. It is used to make soy-free meat alternatives like seitan, and is sometimes nicknamed "wheat meat." The texture and the ability to flavor it in many ways make it a great meat substitute.

**Nutritional yeast (not to be confused with Beer yeast!) can be found in natural foods markets or health food stores, as well as in specialty stores like Trader Joe's. You can also find it in the vegan section or spices section of major supermarkets, as well as in online shops. Nutritional yeast comes as yellowish flakes with a tangy, nutty taste that can be used to make things like cheesy sauces. It can also be sprinkled on top of foods like pasta or margarine toast, as it is a good source of vitamins.

Directions

1. If you are using store-bought vegetable stock, heat the stock in a medium saucepan or boiler until it is hot, but not boiling (the vegetable stock should be hot when used for the recipe).

2. Preheat the oven 375°F.

3. In a large bowl, add the vital wheat gluten, pepper, salt, nutritional yeast, thyme, and paprika and whisk together with a wire whisk or a big fork.

4. Add the olive oil and Bragg's Liquid Aminos (or soy sauce). Then, little by little, pour in the stock (you may not need the whole cup, depending on the gluten you have, so don't pour it all in at once).

5. Mix well with a spoon until the wet ingredients are fully combined with the dry ingredients. Then, work the whole thing into a wet loaf shape with your hand for a few minutes. It should be squishy, but not oozing out liquids. If it's too wet, then add 1 to 3 tablespoons more of the wheat gluten until it gets to that squishy texture.

6. Let the loaf sit for 5 minutes. Then, brush on the molasses (if using). Put the loaf in an oiled casserole dish or a deep pot. Add ½ cup more of stock to keep it from burning and bake for 30 minutes.

7. Once the bottom is cooked, flip the loaf over and bake for an additional 30 minutes. Cut out a small piece to make sure it is fully cooked. Once it is browned and both sides are cooked through, it is ready!

Homemade Seitan Short Ribs in a Bourbon Barbecue Sauce with Sautéed Collards and Tofu Damn Hock Strips

Makes: 4 to 6 servings

Ingredients

Ingredients for Ribs:

2 cups of vital wheat gluten
½ cup of nutritional yeast
¼ cup of **That Ain't NO Hog, Tho: Stanley B Pork Marinade** (See Page 51)
¾ cup of hot vegetable stock + ½ additional cup for baking
1 tablespoon of Bragg's Liquid Aminos
2 tablespoons of olive oil

Ingredients for Collards:

1 bunch of thoroughly-cleaned collard greens, sliced ribbon-style (stack the leaves on top of each other, roll the leaves, and slice across)
2 tablespoons of **That Ain't NO Hog, Tho: Stanley B Pork Marinade**
½ teaspoon of salt
½ teaspoon of pepper

Ingredients for Tofu Hammock Strips:

¼ cup of thinly-sliced tofu marinated in ¼ cup of the **That Ain't NO Hog, Tho: Stanley B Pork Marinade**
1 additional tablespoon of olive oil

Ingredients for Bourbon Barbecue Sauce:

1 cup of good quality ketchup
¼ cup of molasses
½ cup of bourbon (I'm assuming you have it on hand because it goes in a Southern medicine cabinet, but if not, then you can skip it)
2 tablespoons of nutritional yeast
½ teaspoon of sea salt
1 teaspoon of agave (or brown sugar)
1 tablespoon of smoked paprika

Directions

1. Preheat the oven to 400°F. In a large bowl, add the vital wheat gluten and nutritional yeast and whisk together. Next, add in the remaining ingredients and mix lightly with a slotted spoon.

2. Once the liquid starts to mix well with the flour, take the mixture out of the bowl and work the dough with your hands.

3. Stretch out the dough into a flat, rectangular shape and set aside for 5 minutes.

4. Using a small, clean paintbrush or spatula brush, add a little of the faux marinade on the dough and place it in a large, oiled pot or a casserole dish. Pour in ½ cup of vegetable stock in the pot and put the loaf in the oven to bake. Bake for 30 minutes, flip it over and bake for an additional 30 minutes on the other side.

5. While the seitan ribs are baking, make the sauce. In a medium saucepan, add all of the bourbon sauce ingredients EXCEPT the bourbon and whisk them together. Cook over medium-high heat until it starts to bubble slightly. Reduce the heat to medium and add the bourbon. Whisk the bourbon and cook it down until the alcohol has burned off (about 15 minutes).

6. For the collards, heat 1 tablespoon of olive oil in a large skillet over medium heat. Add the marinated tofu "ham" hock strips and lightly fry each side until they have browned.

7. Add the collard greens to a tablespoon of marinade. Sauté the greens for 3-5 minutes. Set aside.

8. Once the seitan rack of ribs has baked, place it on a cutting board. Brush the rack with the bourbon barbecue sauce and slice it into thin, short, rib-shaped pieces.

9. Serve hot, with the greens.

Pea Butter Pesto

The main base of this dish, "pea butter," is a versatile ingredient that can be used in pasta, as a dip with chips, or even as a spread on bread. Let your imagination run wild!

Makes: 2 to 4 servings

Ingredients

2 cups of dry pasta
½ cup o**f Basic Cashew Cream** (See Page 42)
¼ cup diced red onion
1 tablespoon of fresh basil, for garnish

Ingredients for Pea Butter:

1 cup of cooked peas
1 teaspoon of pepper
1 teaspoon of salt
1½ tablespoons of vegan butter
¼ cup of olive oil
2-4 tablespoon of water (as needed, to blend the peas)

Directions

1. Cook the pasta according to the package. Once it is almost fully cooked but still has some bite (al dente), remove from heat. Drain and set aside.

2. Cook the peas until they are very tender (about 3-7 minutes).

3. While they are still hot, add the peas to a blender with salt, pepper, vegan butter, and 1 to 2 tablespoons of water. Blend on a medium speed until everything is well mixed, but not completely smooth.

4. Turn the speed down, unplug the top of the blender, and drizzle in the oil. Mix until the consistency resembles a thick butter.

5. In a large skillet on medium heat, add 1 teaspoon of olive oil and the pasta. Then, add the cashew cream and mix well until it is creamy (like Alfredo sauce).

6. Add the pea butter and red onions and stir with a large, slotted spoon until the pasta is velvety and green.

7. Serve the pasta topped with one tablespoon of fresh, chopped basil as a garnish.

Louisiana-Style Cornmeal-Encrusted Tofu Fish Fry

While growing up, Fridays were Fried Catfish Day. Honestly, although I haven't eaten meat in 15 years (yes, a fish is an animal and therefore, meat!), the one flavor that I do occasionally crave is fish. The now-distant flavor instills memories of popping grease mixed with the sweet sound of soul music and the knowledge that it was about to be the weekend. In my quest to duplicate the textures and flavors reminiscent of those days, I created the following recipe, which infuses sea vegetables with tofu in a Creole spice blend— all wrapped up in a delicious, crunchy batter!

Makes: 3 to 4 servings

Ingredients

1 package of extra-firm tofu
6-8 pieces of dried seaweed, such as nori (find it in the same aisle at the grocery in
   which they have ingredients to make sushi)
¾ cup of cornmeal
½ cup of flour
1½ tablespoon of old bay
½ teaspoon of cumin
1 teaspoon of cayenne
2-3 cups of vegetable oil, for frying

Directions

1. Bring 1-2 cups of water to boil in a small saucepan. Once the water starts to boil, add the seaweed sheets and turn off the heat. While the sheets begin to rehydrate, set them aside.

2. Drain the tofu. Slice the block lengthwise. Cut them into smaller shapes, similar to fish. Using a small paring knife, cut slits or circle shapes in the tofu so that you can insert the seaweed into the slots. Whether cutting slits or circles, **do not pierce all the way through**; otherwise, the seaweed will fall out.

3. In a large bowl, whisk together the flour, spices, and cornmeal.

4. Remove the moist seaweed from the pot and slice it into small pieces. Insert the seaweed pieces into the holes or slits in the tofu.

5. While the tofu is moist, drop it into a large bowl, and coat it completely with the seasoned cornmeal. Flip them over multiple times to fully coat.

6. In a large pot or a fryer, heat the oil to about 400°F. Once the oil is at temperature, drop in the tofu pieces a few at a time, taking care not to overload the pot.

7. Once the pieces are golden on each side (about 2-3 minutes), drain on a plate lined with paper towels.

8. Serve with hot sauce!

Fiya Fiya CamBalaya

Although my Momma is the box food queen (she has always been a working woman), she did introduce me to lots of different flavors, particularly Creole and Cajun. One of those that I really enjoyed was Zatarain's pre-made Jambalaya. You know that commercial, the one with the silhouette playing the jazz clarinet with Nawlins drawl, spiced with Tony Chachere's seasoning! Ooh-wee, damn! I'm getting hungry just thinking about it now! For those of y'all not that familiar with jambalaya, it consists of rice (and not just any rice, but spiced, seasoned, almost dirty rice), red beans, of course, the holy trinity (onion, celery, and bell pepper), and usually 2 or more kinds of meat. This version hits on all of those familiar flavors, and was one of my favorite things to remix! Oh, yeah, and you know it's packing the heat!

Makes: 3 to 4 servings

Ingredients

1 cup of diced **Homemade Seitan** (See Page 150) (You can also use store-bought)
2 cups of cooked wild rice (if using frozen rice, set out to defrost in the fridge or sink)
1 cup of the Holy Trinity: onion, celery, and bell pepper (gotta be green!)
2 garlic cloves, minced
1 cup of cooked red beans
1 teaspoon of sea salt
½ teaspoon of garlic powder
½ teaspoon of pepper
1 minced jalapeño
2 bay leaves
1 tablespoon of hot sauce
1 teaspoon of cayenne
2 tablespoons of olive oil
¼ cup of vegetable stock

Directions

1. In a large skillet (or pot) on medium heat, add the olive oil and sauté the Holy Trinity (onion, bell pepper, and celery) until the onions are translucent and the celery is tender (about 4-6 minutes).

2. Add the seitan, garlic, and jalapeño to brown (about 2-3 minutes). Add the vegetable stock, bay leaves, rice, and all of the spices.

3. Add the beans and stir to mix well. Cook down on a medium heat and simmer for about 15 to 20 minutes, stirring occasionally.

4. Add the hot sauce and let cool. Serve garnished with parsley.

Sesame Rocking Reuben Sandwich

Makes: 2 to 3 sandwiches

Ingredients

8-10 thin slices of **Homemade Seitan** (See Page 150)
4-6 slices of your favorite bread
¼ to ½ cup of shredded cabbage (or sauerkraut)
¼ cup of Russian Sauce*
2 tablespoon of vegan butter

*¼ cup of **Basic Vegan Aioli (Mayo)** (See Page 41) or store-bought vegan mayo, mixed with ¼ cup of diced onion, ¼ cup of ketchup, ¼ cup of diced pickles, and ½ teaspoon of cayenne pepper.

Directions

1. In a large skillet on medium-low heat, melt the vegan butter. Toast the slices of bread until they are golden brown on each side (about 2-4 minutes).

2. Whisk all of the Russian Sauce ingredients together in a medium-sized bowl. Spread one tablespoon of Russian Sauce on each side of the toasted bread.

3. Layer the bread with the sliced seitan and top it with the cabbage/kraut.

4. Serve with "cornichon" or any other type of pickle.

Smoked Baked Macaroni & Cheese

Makes: 4 servings

Ingredients

1 package of rotini pasta (or elbow macaroni)
1 cooked sweet potato
1-2 cups of **Quick, Creamy Cashew Cheese** (See Page 43)
1 teaspoon of pepper
1 teaspoon of liquid smoke
½ teaspoon of smoked paprika
¼ cup of diced tomato, for garnish
1 teaspoon of truffle salt (optional)
Salt & pepper, to taste

Directions

1. Preheat the oven to 375°F.

2. Cook the pasta according to directions. Drain and place in a colander. Rinse under cold water and set aside.

3. Add the sweet potato, cashew cheese, paprika, pepper, and salt to a blender and blend until it is a smooth, cheese consistency.

4. In a large wide casserole pan, add the pasta and cheese sauce. Stir until evenly mixed.

5. Bake in the oven for 20 minutes.

6. Top with the diced tomato and serve.

Tempalo ChickNun Club Salad with Tofu Feta and Vegan Hunty Mustard

This salad eats like a meal! It has salty, savory, sweet, and my favorite spice!

Makes: 2 to 4 servings

Ingredients

½ pack of tempeh, diced into bite-size squares, about the size of dice (I just noticed I talk about dice a lot...mhmmm...)
1 tablespoon of olive oil
½ cup of Louisiana-style hot sauce (or Frank's, if you wanna be bourgeoise about it!)
¼ cup of vegan butter, melted
½ cup of diced tomato
1 bag of mixed greens

Ingredients for Feta:

¼ block of firm tofu
1 tablespoon of lemon juice **or** 1 teaspoon of apple cider vinegar
2 teaspoons of sea salt
1 teaspoon of garlic powder (or 1 garlic clove, finely minced)
1 teaspoon of pepper
2 tablespoons of olive oil
¼ cup of Dijon mustard whisked with 1 tablespoon of agave (or other liquid sweetener), for the dressing

Directions

1. Whisk the hot sauce and vegan butter together in a medium-sized bowl. Set the buffalo sauce aside.

2. Pour the olive oil in a large skillet over medium heat and lightly fry the tempeh bites. Cook them for 2-3 minutes on each side, until they have browned and caramelized. Toss the bites in the bowl of buffalo sauce, making sure to fully coat each bite.

3. Crumble the tofu in a medium-sized bowl until it resembles chunks of feta cheese. Add all of the remaining feta ingredients, saving the olive oil for very last. Mix them with a large spoon.

4. To assemble the salad, place the mixed greens and tomatoes in a large bowl. Pour the dressing around the edges of the bowl in a complete circle. This will ensure that the whole salad gets fully coated and one side won't be too saturated or soggy. Toss with tongs— or your hands, if you ain't afraid to get messy!

5. Add in the buffalo tempeh first, and then the faux feta.

6. If you happen to have any **Rice Paper Bacon BLT** (See Page 190) lying around, crumble it on top!

30-Minute Meals

A common myth with plant-based cooking is that it takes forever to make a meal. I know when I'm talking to my mom on the phone giving her tele-recipes, she always says, "Meme, that sounds like too much work!" Yes, my Momma calls me Meme; don't tell nobody my nickname! Anyway, I know my mom is not alone in feeling that way. While it may take time to create things like seitan from scratch, there are plenty of fun, interesting, and delicious meals you can make that aren't very labor-intense. This section is dedicated to those meals that, even after a long day's work, you won't be too tired to make:

- *Fajita Quesadillas*
- *Mean, Green Nacho Supreme*
- *Blackened Shiitake "Shrimp" over Smoked Kale*
- *Cauliflower Meat*
- *Cauli Jo Burger w/ Blackened Onion*
- *Collard Green-Wrapped Philly Cheese Steak Wraps*
- *Apple-Beer Barbecue Pulled Jackfruit "Pork" Sliders*
- *Portabella Steak Fingers*

C'mon now! I don't wanna hear anybody saying "Ain't nobody got time for that!"

Note: There are three things you will need pre-made for two of the recipes: **Basic Cashew Cream** (See Page 42), **Quick, Creamy Cashew Cheese** (See Page 43), and a frozen bag of rice. If you took my advice in the Tips and Sauce sections (Chapter 4, 5, and 7, respectively), you may already have these in the fridge or freezer, on lock!

Fajita Quesadillas

Makes: 3 to 4 servings

Ingredients

2-3 large Portobello mushroom caps, with the gills removed*
3 multi-colored bell peppers (orange, yellow, red, or whatever you prefer)
½ red onion, sliced into rings (any onion works)
1½ cups of **Quick, Creamy Cashew Cheese** (See Page 43)
2 jalapeños, sliced into long strips
6-8 large tortillas or wraps
¼ cup of olive or vegetable oil
2 tablespoons of store-bought taco seasoning**
½ teaspoon of apple cider vinegar or lemon juice

*If you can't find large ones, then use 1 package of small, de-stemmed mushrooms, such as cremini or button mushrooms.

**Or make your own: 1 teaspoon of cumin, 1 teaspoon of salt, and ½ teaspoon each of garlic powder, chili powder, and paprika.

Directions

1. Preheat oven to the broiler setting.

2. Slice the peppers into long strips or rings and the onion into half-moons, rings, or strips. Slice the mushrooms in ½-inch-thick slices. If you are using the big caps, remove the gills by scraping the underside of the cap with a small spoon.

3. Lay all of the vegetables flat on a cutting board and sprinkle 1 tablespoon of seasoning them.

4. In a large bowl, whisk together the remaining seasoning, the oil, and the lemon juice (or vinegar) into a nice marinade.

5. Add the sliced vegetables into the bowl and toss them using a large spoon (or hands, if you don't mind getting a little nitty-gritty).

6. Make sure the veggies are fully coated with the marinade and then lay them flat onto a slightly-oiled baking sheet. Place the baking sheet into the broiler to char. **Note:** It is important to check them every 2-3 minutes, because the broiler is intense and will incinerate them quickly!

7. Warm the tortilla shells. My preferred method is to lay them directly on the burner (if you have a gas stove) for a few seconds on each side to char. However, you can also place them directly on your oven racks, making sure the broiler is off.

8. Assemble the quesadillas by smearing a generous amount of the **Creamy Cashew Cheese** on the tortilla. Then, spread a handful of the veggies evenly throughout the tortilla to cover the surface. Take another shell and spread more creamy cheese to one side of it. Place this on top of the veggie-covered surface (sandwich-style.) Repeat with the remaining ingredients.

9. Using a sharp knife or a pizza cutter, slice the quesadilla in half vertically. Then, slice it in half horizontally. You should have 4 equally-sized, triangular-shaped slices. Repeat with all of the quesadillas.

10. Top with your favorite salsa, hot sauce, or more of the **Creamy Cashew Cheese.**

Mean, Green Nacho Supreme

Makes: 2 to 4 servings

Ingredients

1 bag blue corn tortilla chips (any tortilla chips will do)
1 can of black beans, cooked
1 bunch of spinach or kale
½ teaspoon of salt
1 teaspoon of garlic powder
1 cup of diced tomato
½ cup of diced onion
1 diced jalapeño
¼ cup of minced cilantro **or** ½ teaspoon of coriander powder
1 cup of sliced sautéed mushrooms
2 teaspoons of taco seasoning
4 tablespoons of olive oil
½ cup of sliced olives (optional)

Ingredients for Avocado Crema:

1 pitted avocado
1 cup of **Quick, Creamy Cashew Cheese** (See Page 43)
½ teaspoon of sea salt
½ teaspoon of black pepper
½ teaspoon of garlic powder
½ to 1 cup of water
Juice of 1 lime (optional, but highly recommended!)

Directions

<u>For the Crema</u>

1.   In a blender, add ½ cup of water. Next, add the remaining ingredients and blend on a medium speed. You want it to be creamy and the consistency of nacho cheese (only this one will be green!). If it is too thick, blend again with an additional ½ cup of water.

2.   Set aside.

<u>For the Nachos</u>

1.   In a large bowl, add the diced tomato, onion, cilantro, jalapeño, lime juice (if using) and a pinch of salt. Stir with a large spoon. Set the quick pico aside.

2. Place the canned beans into a medium-sized saucepan. Add 1 teaspoon of the taco seasoning and cook the beans.

3. Heat 1 tablespoon of olive oil in a medium-sized skillet over medium heat. Place the sliced mushrooms onto a cutting board. Sprinkle the remaining teaspoon of taco seasoning onto the mushrooms. Add them to the skillet and sauté until they're tender (about 3-5 minutes). Remove the mushrooms and set aside.

4. Add another tablespoon of olive oil and the greens to the same skillet. Sprinkle on the garlic powder and sea salt and sauté them over medium heat until wilted, but not soggy (about 2-5 minutes).

5. To assemble the nachos, on a large plate or serving platter, arrange the chips in a circle.

   Tip: heat the chips for 2-3 minutes on a baking sheet in the oven preheated to 375°F.

6. Place the beans evenly along the ring of chips. Next, spread the mushrooms along the ring, over the beans. Then, spread the greens evenly across the mushrooms. Spread the salsa on top of the greens. Top the nachos off by drizzling the crema along the ring with a spoon. If you wanna be fancy, fill a squeeze bottle with the crema and drizzle with that, instead.

7. If using, then top with sliced olives and serve.

Blackened Shiitake "Shrimp" over Smoked Kale

Nothing spells Southern like blackened and charred food. Burn a little toast, and we call it Cajun-style. One of my favorite ways to impart flavor into foods is by blackening them. This technique has roots in the bayous of Louisiana. It allows you to get flavoring from the seasonings that sticks to the food. With flexible texture and rich earthiness, shiitake mushrooms make the perfect substitute for shrimp in this Cajun treat!

Makes: 2 servings

Ingredients
1 package of fresh shiitake mushrooms (8-10 ounces)
2 tablespoon of vegan butter (you can use olive oil instead, if you prefer)
1½ tablespoons of blackening spice *
3 cups of kale (or another sturdy green, such as chard or collard green)
1 teaspoon of liquid smoke
3 garlic cloves, sliced
1 tablespoon of olive oil

*Blackening spice a blend of cayenne pepper, garlic powder, paprika, salt, pepper, thyme, which can be found in the spices section of grocery stores

Directions

1. Heat a well-oiled, seasoned cast iron skillet over medium heat for 5-7 minutes. If it starts to smoke heavily, then lower the heat slightly.

2. With a pair of scissors or kitchen shears, cut off the stems of the shiitake mushrooms, leaving only the caps. Save the stems for making vegetable stock. Using a small paring knife, cut the caps into a curved, shrimp-like shape.

3. In a small pot, melt the vegan butter. Set aside.

4. Pour the blackened seasoning into a bowl. Dip the cleaned shiitake "shrimp" in the hot vegan butter first, then into the blackening rub, making sure to coat each side while pressing down onto the hot cast iron skillet.

5. Using a spatula or fork, press the "shrimp" down hard on the pan to sear (you should hear a sizzle). Let them stick for a minute or two to blacken. Lift up a corner of one to make sure it has a dark, caramelized color before flipping it over to brown the other side. Repeat for all of the "shrimp." Drain on a napkin-lined plate.

6. In a separate skillet, heat the additional tablespoon of olive oil and garlic on medium heat. Add the kale (or other sturdy green) to the pan. Pour the liquid smoke onto the green and sauté until the leaves wilt (about 1-2 minutes). Turn off the heat and let greens continue to cook in the residual heat.

7. Serve the shiitake over the green and top with some good ole Louisiana-Style Hot Sauce.

Cauliflower Meat

Cauliflower is quickly turning into the vegan world's "IT" gurl! It's so fabulous, how can it *not* be?! As you may have noticed by now, I love to repurpose and transform produce into all kinds of new, inventive creations. One new use that I've found for cauliflower is to turn it into a "meat." I found this out during a month of a raw-food diet. Cauliflower is so dope not only for its blank canvas status, but also because it's super low-calorie. You can use the "meat" for tacos, spaghetti, and even burritos!

Makes: 4 servings

Ingredients

1 head of cauliflower
1 ripe tomato
3 tablespoons of olive oil
1 garlic clove
¼ cup of diced onion
1 teaspoon of salt
1 teaspoon of pepper
1 teaspoon of cumin
1 teaspoon of chili powder
1 teaspoon of garlic powder

Directions

1. In a dry blender or a food processor, pulse the cauliflower for a few seconds to break it down slightly.

2. Add the tomato, spices, seasonings, and 2 of the 3 tablespoons of olive oil, and pulse again on a medium speed for about 5-10 seconds.

3. In a large skillet, pour in the remaining tablespoon of olive oil and onions. Sauté them on medium heat for about 3 minutes.

4. Once the onions have started to *sweat* (release water), add the cauliflower meat mixture.

5. Stir the mixture in with the onions and brown until it is a taco meat consistency (about 3 minutes).

6. Taste and adjust the flavor with salt and pepper, if desired.

Cauli Jo Burger w/ Blackened Onion

Makes: 2 to 4 burgers

Ingredients

2-8 slices of your favorite bread or 2-4 burger buns
Cauliflower Meat (See previous recipe)
1 FLEGG (1 tablespoon dissolved in 3 tablespoons of warm water)
2 tablespoons of tomato paste
1 large, red onion, sliced into rings
2 tablespoons of olive oil
1 teaspoon of sea salt

Directions

1. Make the FLEGG and set it aside for 10 minutes, until it is a gluey consistency.

2. Heat a well-seasoned cast iron skillet on medium heat.

3. Add the cooked cauliflower meat, tomato paste, and FLEGG to the skillet and mix with a large spoon. Next, form the mixture into medium-sized patties resembling hamburger patties. Set aside on a plate.

4. Toss the red onion in a bowl with the salt, pepper, and 1 tablespoon of olive oil. Place the onions in the cast iron skillet and press down with a spatula, allowing them to sear and blacken (about 2-3 minutes on each side). Set on a plate lined with a napkin to cool.

5. Pour the last tablespoon of olive oil in the cast iron skillet, and place the patties into the skillet, pressing down firmly with the spatula. Since the "meat" is pre-cooked, this is just to get a bit of crispness on each side. Cook for about 3 minutes on each side.

6. Serve the Cauli Jo Burgers on a toasted bun with the blackened onion for a nice depth of flavor. Save any remaining onions for a spread.

Collard Green-Wrapped Philly Cheese Steak Wraps

This dish definitely reps a bit of my journey from my Southern roots to my East Coast development as a cook. One of my favorite cities in the US is Philadelphia, and this is my shout out to the city that has shown me nuthin' but love.

Makes: 2 to 4 servings

Ingredients

5 large collard green leaves, washed and de-stemmed
1-2 cups of ice mixed with 1 cup of cold water
2 large Portobello mushroom caps sliced thinly
¼ cup of olive oil
½ cup onion, sliced thinly and sautéed
1 teaspoon of cumin
1 teaspoon of Bragg's Liquid Aminos
2 tablespoons of balsamic vinegar

Ingredients for Cheese Sauce:

2 cups of cooked sweet potato
1 tablespoon of apple cider vinegar
¼ cup of nutritional yeast
1 tablespoon of garlic powder
¼ cup of olive oil

Directions

1. In a large pot, bring 2 cups of water to boil. In a separate bowl, mix the ice and the water and set aside, near the pot.

2. Clean the collard green leaf, and break off the bottom part of the stem. Make sure to keep the collard leaf intact. Once the water in the pot is boiling, drop in the leaves and blanch for about 1-2 minutes, then immediately remove the leaves from the pot with tongs and shock them in the bowl of ice (also known as an *ice bath*). Set aside.

3. Make the cheese sauce by adding all of the ingredients (sweet potato, apple cider vinegar, nutritional yeast, and garlic powder) **EXCEPT** the olive oil to the blender. Blend on medium until smooth. Once they are fully mixed, drop the blender speed down to low. Unplug the top of the blender and slowly drizzle in the olive oil. Set aside.

4. In a large skillet, add in the olive oil, portabella mushroom slices, and onions and sauté for about 3-5 minutes. Add the cumin and Bragg's and cook down until the mushrooms are fully cooked and browned (about 3-5 minutes).

5. In a medium saucepan, heat the cheese mixture for 3-5 minutes or until it is bubbling.

6. To assemble the wraps, drain the collard leaves and lay them flat on a cutting board. Fill the leaf down the middle with mushrooms and onions. Take a large spoon and drizzle in the cheese.

7. Take the bottom of the leaf and fold up. Then, while holding the bottom, fold in the left and right sides, like a burrito. Roll all the way up to secure the wraps. To make it extra indulgent, drizzle more cheese on top!

Apple-Beer Barbecue Pulled Jackfruit "Pork" Sliders

Makes: 2 to 4 servings

Ingredients

4 Brioche buns (or any small buns)
2 cans of jackfruit in brine water (NOT syrup) **OR** artichoke hearts (pulled apart and chopped until they resemble pulled meat)
4 thickly-sliced red onions
1 tablespoon of olive oil, to toast the buns

Ingredients for Marinade:

¼ cup of olive oil
2 teaspoons of sea salt
2 tablespoons of almond butter (or peanut butter)
1 tablespoon of nutritional yeast
1 tablespoon of apple cider vinegar

Ingredients for BBQ Sauce:

½ cup of apple-flavored beer (can you substitute ginger beer for a non-alcoholic version)
1 cup of ketchup
1 teaspoon of liquid smoke
2 tablespoons of molasses
1 teaspoon of cayenne

Directions

1. In a large bowl, whisk together all of the marinade ingredients and set aside.

2. Drain the jackfruit, take it apart, and remove the seeds. You should have a stringy texture. Place the jackfruit "pork" in the marinade bowl and set aside.

3. In a large saucepan, whisk all of the barbecue sauce ingredients together. Bring to a boil.

4. Once it starts to boil and most of the liquid has evaporated, reduce to a low simmer and add in the jackfruit pork.

5. Braise the pork in the sauce for about 15 minutes.

6. To assemble the sliders, cut the buns in half and toast them in a large skillet with olive oil over medium-to-high heat (about 2-3 minutes).

7. Add the pork and top with thickly-sliced onions.

Portabella Steak Fingers

Whenever my family and I would take trips from Houston to the country to visit my grandma, we would always stop in this small town called Hearne, about 30 minutes from our destination, to visit a Dairy Queen. The first step in my plant-based journey was cutting out red meat, around the age of 12. So instead of burgers, I'd always get the chicken-fried steak-finger basket. Looking back, I'm really not sure what they were, but, if I had to guess, I'd say it was actually some type of ground beef-like thing battered and country-fried. It was always served with Texas toast and gravy, with a red-checkered paper lining the box. The beefy-ness in this recipe provides that same texture, and at least we know what's in this one!

Makes: 3 to 4 servings

Ingredients

3-4 large Portabella mushroom caps
1 cup of flour seasoned with 1 tablespoon each of salt, pepper, and cayenne
1-2 cups of vegetable oil, for frying

Ingredients for Steak Marinade:

¼ cup of balsamic vinegar
½ cup of olive oil or other mild oil
1 teaspoon of salt
1 teaspoon of cumin
1 teaspoon of pepper
1 teaspoon of agave syrup (or similar liquid sweetener)
1 tablespoon of nutritional yeast (optional)
½ teaspoon of cayenne pepper (optional)

Directions

1. In a large bowl, whisk together all of the marinade ingredients.

2. Clean the gills from the mushroom (by scrapping the inside of the cap with a spoon) and remove the stems. Save these for gravies or stock. Wipe off the mushroom caps with a damp napkin or a vegetable brush.

3. Cut the caps into thirds, until you have thick, long strips. Toss the strips in the marinade and fully coat each strip. Let them sit while you heat the oil.

4. Heat the vegetable oil in a deep saucepan or a fryer until it reaches between 385 and 400°F.

5. Pour the seasoned flour in a medium-sized plastic bag. Once the oil is at temperature, dredge the strips in the flour bag and shake them.

6. Drop the strips, gently, into the hot oil and fry on each side until golden brown (about 2-5 minutes).

7. Drain on a plate lined with a paper towel.

Tip: This also tastes great with my **Mushroom Gravy** (See Page 122).

Kitchen Aces

Where all my kitchen aces at? Maybe you've been around the vegan block for a while, or maybe you have that "been there, done that" attitude with plant-based cookbooks? Or, even better, maybe you want to practice for your upcoming Chopped episode? This section has recipes that are little more labor-intensive, but well worth the effort:

- *Eggplant Phish Sticks*
- *Cauliflower 'Chicken' with Stewed Okra and Tomato*
- *Cremini & Farro Swedish Meatballs*
- *Blackened Spice-Crusted Whole Cauliflower Head*
- *Tempeh Boudin Balls, Y'all*
- *Rice Paper Bacon BLT w/ Caramelized Onion Mayo*
- *Carrie B's Cornbread Dressing*
- *Fall Vegetable & Wild Rice Dressing with Wild Mushroom Red-Eye Gravy*
- *A Texan in Italy: Fried Green Tomato Caprese Salad*
- *Garlicky Shrimp & Grits*
- *Stuffed Acorn Squash with Blackened Kale*
- *Palm Po' Boy with Creamy Cocktail Sauce*

Give these a try, and wow your family!

Eggplant Phish Sticks

Makes: 3 to 4 servings

Ingredients

2 medium-sized eggplants
1½ cups of all-purpose flour
1 cup of nondairy milk + 1 tablespoon of apple cider vinegar
1 cup of finely-minced seaweed snacks **or** 1 tablespoon of dulse flakes
1½ tablespoons of old bay seasoning
¼ cup of olive oil
1 tablespoon of lemon juice
1 cup of panko bread crumbs
Enough oil to cover the sticks for frying (this will depend on the size of your pot)
Salt and pepper, to taste (optional; about ½ teaspoon each, if using)

Directions

1. Mince the seaweed snacks into fine pieces. Put them in a large bowl and whisk-in the lemon juice and olive oil. Set marinade aside.

2. Cut off the ends of the eggplant, so that it stands up on the cutting board. Cut the eggplant in half, lengthwise. Then, cut each half into a long spear or stick. They should be ½- to ¾-inches thick.

3. Set eggplant sticks in the marinade and set aside.

4. In a deep pot or a fryer, pour in the cooking oil, about 4-6 inches high. You should have enough to completely cover the top of the sticks. While the oil is getting to temperature (between 385 and 400°F), set up your breading station.

5. Get three bowls for the set-up and add the following to each:

   -For the first bowl, add 1 cup of flour.
   -For the middle bowl, add the cup of milk-and-vinegar mixture.
   -In the last bowl, add 1 cup of panko mixed with the remaining tablespoon of old bay.

6. Once the oil reaches temperature and it is bubbling (but not smoking), it is ready for frying. Remove a stick from the marinade and coat it in the 1st bowl of flour. Next, dip it into the liquid bowl, and finally, the 3rd bowl of seasoned panko. Now, place it in the fryer. Repeat this process with the remaining sticks, being careful not to overcrowd the pot.

7. Using tongs or a metal, slotted spoon, fry the sticks until they are golden on each side and crispy (about 2-5 minutes). You don't want them to soak up too much oil and get soggy, so don't leave them in for too long! Place them on a plate lined with a paper towel.

8. Serve them while they are hot!

Tip: This recipe goes well with the extra **Creamy Cocktail Sauce** (See Page 200).

Cauliflower 'Chicken' with Stewed Okra and Tomato

Although my momma wasn't one to spend hours slaving in the kitchen, one homemade dish that she made, which was full of love and soul, was a big pot of stewed okra and tomato with chicken-on-the-bone. This was the kind of dish that made your whole house smell like love. It had that feel of comfort when you know somebody had been in the kitchen all day, even though it didn't take that long to make. Although I don't eat chicken anymore, I'm still able to get this same warm and fuzzy realness by using cauliflower chicken! Cooking the cauliflower separately and later adding it to the stew creates that a fried chickeny flavor typical of this dish.

Makes: 3 to 4 servings

Ingredients

1 head of cauliflower, broken into large florets (you can buy it already broken; I just prefer the head so I can use it for multiple purposes)
2 cups vegetable oil, for frying
1 cup of flour
2 tablespoon of poultry seasoning*
1 package of fresh okra (about 15-18 pieces), sliced in half, lengthwise (you can substitute frozen, if needed)
2 large, ripe tomatoes, medium-diced
¼ cup of diced onions
2 tablespoons of minced garlic
2 tablespoons of olive oil
1 cup of vegetable stock
1 teaspoon of salt
1 teaspoon of pepper

*Or make your own, using ½ teaspoon each of paprika, sage, salt, pepper, and garlic powder.

Directions

1. Season the cauliflower florets thoroughly with the poultry seasoning. Pour the flour into a plastic bag.

2. Heat the frying oil in a medium to large saucepan or fryer.

3. In a separate, large stock pot*, add the olive oil and brown the onion and garlic for about 2 to 4 minutes. Pour in the vegetable stock to *deglaze* (prevent from sticking) and add the tomato and okra. Cook uncovered on medium heat for about 3-5 minutes so the tomato and okra start to break down.

4. Once the oil is hot, place the cauliflower in the plastic bag of flour and shake to lightly bread the cauliflower.

5. When the oil is around 350 to 375°F, add the breaded cauliflower to fry.

6. Once the cauliflower is browned on each side (about 2-5 minutes), add the cauliflower "chicken" to the pot of stew and mix with a large spoon.

7. Simmer on medium-to-low heat for 15 to 20 minutes, until everything is tender. The tomatoes should become broken down, and all of the ingredients should become incorporated together into a nice stew.

8. Taste and add salt and pepper, if necessary. Serve alone or with rice.

*A stock pot is a deep pot, usually with handles, that is usually used to make soups or stews.

Cremini & Farro Swedish Meatballs

Makes: 4 to 6 servings

Ingredients

1 cup of farro, cooked (you can use brown rice instead as your binder, but farro works better!)
1 10-ounce pack of cremini or button mushrooms (12-14 mushrooms)
1½ cups of breadcrumbs
1 medium-sized tomato, diced
2 tablespoons of olive oil
1 teaspoon of finely-chopped fennel seed (you can also use ground)
1 tablespoon of cumin
1-2 teaspoons of salt
½ teaspoon of pepper
1 teaspoon of garlic powder
2 tablespoons of ground flaxseed mixed with 4 tablespoons of warm water, to make FLEGG*
1 teaspoon of steak seasoning (optional)

*Let it sit until it is a gluey texture while you are preparing the other ingredients. It usually takes around 5 to 7 minutes to turn gluey. If it separates, mix it with a fork.

Directions

1. Preheat the oven to 400°F.

2. In a large bowl, toss the cleaned mushroom caps with 1 tablespoon of olive oil and 1 teaspoon of salt and pepper.

3. In a medium-to-large skillet, add 1 tablespoon of olive oil and sauté the seasoned mushrooms until tender (about 3-5 minutes). Don't overload the pan with mushrooms!

4. Add the tomato and mushrooms into a blender and pulse on a medium speed for a few seconds, just to breakdown.

5. In a large bowl, add the mushroom-tomato mixture, the farro, breadcrumbs, FLEGG, and all of the other ingredients and seasonings. Stir with a large spoon.

6. With your hands, form the mixture into meatballs and place them onto an oiled baking sheet. If you are having trouble getting them to bind, add more breadcrumbs, ¼ cup at a time.

7. Drizzle a little olive oil on the tops of each meatball and bake in the oven for 15 to 20 minutes. Break one to test if they are done. Flip the meatballs over and bake for another 8 to 10 minutes before serving.

Blackened Spice-Crusted Whole Cauliflower Head

Makes: 3 to 4 servings

Ingredients

1 large head of cauliflower
1 cup of **Basic Cashew Cream** (See Page 42) + 2 tablespoons of apple cider vinegar
2 tablespoons of cayenne blackening blend*
2 tablespoons of olive oil

*If you are making the blend from scratch, then use ¼ teaspoon each of sage, thyme, paprika, cayenne, garlic powder, and pepper, plus 1 teaspoon of sea salt.

Directions

1. Preheat the oven 400°F.

2. Clean the cauliflower head by removing the green leaves and thick, inedible stems carefully, keeping the head intact.

3. In a large bowl, whisk the curdled cashew cream and spice blend until it is well mixed.

4. Completely coat the cauliflower head with the spice spread using a brush or a spatula (although, I prefer getting down and dirty and using my hands!).

5. Drizzle the olive oil over the cauliflower head.

6. Place the cauliflower head in an oiled, deep pan or casserole dish and roast for 45 to 60 minutes, or until it is fully cooked. Ideally, you want a crust, browning on the edges, and a tender yet slightly firm consistency.

7. Serve as the main centerpiece by cutting the head into thick wedges. Use the leftover spread for a dip.

Tempeh Boudin Balls, Y'all

Boudin balls are arguably the quintessential Creole classic. Everybody's auntie has their own spin on these, ranging from the types and parts of meat that are stuffed in them to the shape. They are also served for breakfast or as a side with gumbo. I wanted to find a way to duplicate the sausage encasing that is authentic to this dish, and I found it with rice paper. So, as they say in Nawlins, "laissez-faire!"

Makes: 3 to 4 servings

Ingredients

1½ cups of rice, cooked
8-10 sheets of rice paper
½ cup of diced Holy Trinity (onion, bell pepper, and celery)
1 jalapeño, minced
1 tablespoon of olive oil
2 cups of vegetable oil, for frying

Ingredients for Tempeh Pork Marinade:

1 block of tempeh
½ cup of olive oil
1 tablespoon of salt
1 tablespoon of nutritional yeast
1 tablespoon of apple cider vinegar
1½ tablespoons of nut butter (peanut or almond)
1 teaspoon of garlic powder
1 teaspoon of paprika
1 teaspoon of cayenne

Directions

1. In a large bowl, whisk together all of the marinade ingredients **EXCEPT** the tempeh.

2. Crumble the tempeh into the marinade and stir it with a large spoon. Set aside.

3. In a large skillet, heat 1 tablespoon of olive oil and sauté the Holy Trinity ingredients until they are slightly browned (about 2-4 minutes).

4. Stir in the rice and the jalapeño until fully incorporated and cooked. Add the tempeh to the skillet and stir the mixture together to mix well. Set aside.

5. Fill a large bowl with water and add 1 sheet of rice paper to rehydrate it for 5-10 seconds. Remove the sheet and place it on a cutting board.

6. Using a spoon or a small scooper, scoop out the rice tempeh mixture and put it on the hydrated rice paper sheet. Pulling the paper tight, roll up the paper to create a rice mixture-filled ball.

7. Repeat this with all of the remaining sheets of rice paper until the whole rice mixture is used.

8. Set the balls on a baking sheet to dry in the oven while the oil is heating.

9. In a large pot or a fryer, heat the vegetable oil to 375°F. Once the oil is at temperature, drop the balls into the pot, taking care not to overcrowd the pot, and fry them.

10. Turn them over to get all of the sides golden brown (about 1-3 minutes per side). Drain on a plate lined with a napkin.

Rice Paper Bacon BLT w/ Caramelized Onion Mayo

Anybody from the South knows that pork makes part of almost all meals! Having grown up with those types of meals as part of my roots, I'm always looking for ways to create bacon out of something. This recipe features one of the most convincing mock bacons I've ever made. Using rice paper, this recipe gets that nice crispiness that works so well in a bacon-filled sandwich. I would suggest making double, because it ain't gonna last long!

Makes: 2 sandwiches

Ingredients

Ingredients for Bacon (in this case, "facon!"):

6 sheets of rice paper
1 cup of water
1 cup of ***That Ain't NO Hog, Tho: Stanley B Pork Marinade*** (See Page 51)

Ingredients for Caramelized Onion Mayo:

1 cup of caramelized onion
1 cup of **Basic Vegan Aioli (Mayo)** (See Page 41), or store-bought vegan mayo

Additional Toppings

1 sliced tomato
4-5 fresh lettuce leaves
4 pieces of your favorite bread, toasted

Directions

1. Preheat the oven to 375°F.

2. Stack the sheets on top of each other, two at a time, and cut them into strips.

3. In a large bowl, pour in the faux pork marinade. In another bowl, add one cup of water.

4. Dip the strips in the water bowl for about 10 seconds to soften. Squeeze out the residual water.

5. Dunk the strips in the marinade. Completely cover each side with the marinade. Lay flat on a baking sheet lined with parchment paper, if you have it, or a well-oiled sheet.

6. Bake until the strips are crisp on each side and no longer wet (about 20-25 minutes on each side).

7. While the facon bakes, whip up the mayo. Add the caramelized onion and aioli into a blender and blend on medium speed for about 20 to 30 seconds.

8. To serve, smear on the mayo on each side of the toast, then add the lettuce and tomato, and top with the rice paper bacon.

Carrie B's Cornbread Dressing

The most asked question when it comes to where you are spending the holidays in the South is, "Who gone make the dressing?" For those of y'all not fluent in Southern, dressing is stuffing...and I ain't talking 'bout Stovetop. I knew it was gonna be a good holiday if that dressing was made by my momma. Her dressing was so good, you didn't even need that congealed cranberry sauce! This is my ode to my momma's dressing, sans the hardboiled egg!

Makes: 3 to 4 servings

Ingredients

Ingredients for Cornbread:

1 cup of cornmeal
1 cup of flour
3 teaspoons of baking powder
2 tablespoons of sugar
1 teaspoon of salt
¼ cup vegetable oil
1 cup of nondairy milk mixed with 1 tablespoon of apple cider vinegar
2 tablespoons of FLEGG (1 tablespoon of ground flaxseed + 2 tablespoons of warm water)

Ingredients for Dressing:

1 cup of cooked, diced **Homemade Seitan** (See Page 150) (this is optional if you don't already have it on hand, but is recommended; you can substitute with diced store-bought as well.)
¼ cup of diced celery
¼ of an onion, diced
¼ of a green pepper, diced
½ cup of vegetable stock
1 teaspoon of salt
1 teaspoon of pepper
1 teaspoon of cayenne
1 teaspoon of thyme
1 teaspoon of sage

Directions

1. Preheat the oven to 400°F. In a small bowl, mix up the ingredients to make FLEGG and let it sit for about 10 minutes (remember that 'gluey' consistency you want it to have).

2. In another small bowl, mix the apple cider vinegar with the nondairy milk to make buttermilk.

3. In a large bowl, whisk together all of the dry cornbread ingredients. Then add the milk, oil, and FLEGG, and stir them together with a large spoon until it forms a batter.

4. Pour the batter into a well-oiled, seasoned cast-iron skillet and bake until fully cooked (about 17 to 20 minutes).

5. Once the cornbread is fully cooked, crumble it in a large bowl.

6. Add in all of the remaining ingredients (vegetables, seitan, and spices) and stir. Pour in the vegetable stock ¼ cup at a time and mix until it's very moist.

7. Put the mixture back into the pan or casserole dish and bake until it has dried out somewhat and is fluffy (around 20 minutes).

8. Cool for 5 minutes and serve.

Fall Vegetable & Wild Rice Dressing with Wild Mushroom Red-Eye Gravy

Makes: 3 to 4 servings

Ingredients

3 cups of cornbread (As prepared in the previous recipe)
½ cup of vegetable stock
1 ½ cups of cooked wild rice (If you are using rice from a previously frozen batch, then let it defrost slightly in the fridge or on the counter over a plate for draining)
1 cup of chopped squash or pumpkin
1 cup of chopped fresh kale (or preferred green)
1 teaspoon of salt
1 teaspoon of pepper
1 teaspoon of cayenne
1 teaspoon of thyme
1 teaspoon of sage

Ingredients for Gravy:

1-cup of wild mushroom and scraps that you may have left over from mushroom stems, stocks or other dishes
1 cup of flour
½ to 1 cup of prepared coffee (as needed)
½ cup of diced onion
1 teaspoon of salt
1 teaspoon of pepper
¼ cup of olive oil
1 tablespoon of arrowroot/cornstarch + 3 tablespoons water (optional for thicker gravy)

Directions

1. Preheat the oven to 400°F.

2. Crumble the fully-cooked cornbread in a large bowl. Add all of the remaining dressing ingredients **EXCEPT** for the stock, and mix them together with a large spoon.

3. Slowly add the vegetable stock ½ cup at a time, until the dressing is a wet and has a somewhat sticky consistency.

4. Pour the dressing mixture into a well-seasoned cast iron skillet or casserole dish. Bake in the oven for about 20 to 30 minutes, until it has dried out somewhat and is fluffy.

5. While the dressing is baking, prepare the red-eye gravy. Heat the oil in a large skillet over medium heat and sauté the mushrooms and onions until they are slightly browned (about 2-4 minutes).

6. Add the flour to the oil and whisk lightly. The flour will turn into a thick, dark roux and will stick to the whisk. Pour in the coffee and whisk the roux to thin it out. Then, whisk it vigorously until it gets to a gravy consistency. Pour in the salt and pepper and continue to whisk.

7. **If you prefer thicker gravy,** then add an arrowroot/cornstarch "slurry" to the gravy pan. To make slurry, mix 1 tablespoon of arrowroot/cornstarch with 3 tablespoons of water and whisk together; the mixture should have the consistency of coffee creamer.

8. **If you prefer thinner gravy,** thin out the gravy with more stock, a few tablespoons at a time.

9. Ladle the gravy over a big old heaping bowl of the dressing!

A Texan in Italy: Fried Green Tomato Caprese Salad

Makes: 2 servings

Ingredients

4 firm green tomatoes
1 teaspoon of old bay seasoning
1 cup of flour + 1 teaspoon of old bay seasoning
1 cup of nondairy milk mixed with 1 tablespoon of apple cider vinegar
1 cup of seasoned panko breadcrumbs
1 cup of **Quick, Creamy Cashew Cheese** (See Page 43)
4 basil leaves, flash-fried in vegetable oil for a few seconds
1 cup of panko seasoned with 1 teaspoon of salt and pepper blend

Ingredients for Tomato Jam:

4 ripe tomatoes
1 onion, diced
2 garlic cloves
1 tablespoon of molasses
½ to 1 teaspoon of liquid smoke
2-3 teaspoons of miso paste (think sushi isle at the grocery store)
2 tablespoons of olive oil

Ingredients for Balsamic Reduction:

1 cup of balsamic vinegar

Directions

For Jam

1. In a large stock pot, sauté the onions and garlic in olive oil.

2. Add the tomatoes to a blender and pulse on a medium speed for 5 to 10 seconds. Pour into the pot.

3. Add all the remaining jam ingredients to the pot and stir to fully incorporate.

4. Reduce the temperature to a medium low temperature and simmer uncovered until most of the liquid has evaporated and it takes on a jam-like consistency (about 25-30 minutes).

For Balsamic Reduction

1. Heat 1 cup of balsamic vinegar on medium high until it starts to boil. Make sure you have a window open or your exhaust fan on, as the low fumes may get to you.

2. Once it has started to boil, reduce to a low simmer for 7 to 10 minutes stirring it somewhat often until the consistency is slightly syrupy and coats the spoon when you stick it in. Set aside.

For Fried Green Tomatoes

1. Rinse off the tomatoes and cut them into ½-inch-thick slices.

2. Season the slices with the old bay seasoning.

3. In a small bowl, mix the milk with the apple cider vinegar to make buttermilk.

4. In a large pot or fryer, heat the vegetable oil until it reaches 400°F.

5. Set up a breading station by taking a bowl of panko crumbs, a bowl of seasoned flour, and the bowl of buttermilk.

6. Dip a slice of tomato in the flour, then the buttermilk, and lastly, in the panko, making sure it's fully coated. Repeat with all of the tomato slices.

7. Once the oil is at temperature (around 375°F), slightly drop in the breaded tomato slices, careful not to overcrowd the pot. Fry on each side until golden brown (about 2-3 minutes). Drain on a plate lined with a paper towel. Turn off the heat.

8. While the grease is cooling, drop a few basil leaves in for a few seconds to crisp them.

To Assemble the Caprese Salad:

1. Lay a slice of fried tomato on the center of the plate. Place a scoop of the jam on one side and the cashew cheese on the other.

2. Drizzle the balsamic reduction around the plate.

3. Garnish the tomato with a crispy basil leaf.

Garlicky Shrimp & Grits

Warning: You may not want to kiss nobody after this dish! If you aren't a garlic fan, then skip this one altogether. If you dare try it, it's definitely a good one!

Makes: 2 servings

Ingredients

2 large heads of garlic
¼ olive oil
1 teaspoon dulse flakes*
1 tablespoon of old bay seasoning
1 teaspoon of thyme
¼ cup of beet juice
1 cup of polenta
1 cup of vegetable stock

*If you can't find these, mince ½ cup of seaweed sheet snacks
  for that seafood flavor.

Directions

1. In a large bowl, mix the olive oil, thyme, beet juice, old bay seasoning, Dulse flakes, and salt together. Set aside.

2. Remove the bottom core from each garlic head, but leave the rest of them intact.

3. Place the garlic heads in a large pot of boiling water and boil until tender (about 10 to 15 minutes). Place the garlic in the marinade and set aside.

4. Bring 1 cup of vegetable stock to boil in a medium-sized saucepan. Reduce the temperate and slowly add the polenta while whisking it (*very* slowly, so it doesn't boil over!). Keep the pan on a low heat.

5. Heat a cast-iron skillet over medium heat for about 5 minutes.

6. Pour 1 tablespoon of olive oil in the pan and add the garlic shrimp. Press down with a spatula and sear each side for about 3-5 minutes.

7. Serve on top of the polenta.

Stuffed Acorn Squash with Blackened Kale

Makes: 4 servings

Ingredients

2 whole acorn squash
1 hunk of stale bread
1 teaspoon each of sage, thyme, and garlic powder
1 teaspoon of salt
2 cups of kale (you can substitute the kale with collard or mustard greens)
2 garlic cloves, sliced
2 tablespoon of olive oil

Directions

1. Preheat the oven to 375°F. Slice each squash in half and scoop out the middle.

2. Drizzle 1 tablespoon of olive oil into each squash and dust with 1 teaspoon of salt and pepper.

3. Place face-down on a baking sheet and place in the oven. Bake for 20 minutes.

4. In a large skillet, heat 1 tablespoon of olive oil and add the kale (or green of choice) and garlic. Let it stick. Then add the cubed bread, the rest of the spices, and ¼ cup of stock.

5. Mix well and cook for 3- 5 minutes.

6. Using a large spoon, scoop the stuffing into the squash and bake for an additional 30 minutes or until the mixture isn't wet and the squash is tender.

Palm Po' Boy with Creamy Cocktail Sauce

Makes: 2 to 4 sandwiches

Ingredients

2 large baguettes
2 cans of hearts of palm (if you can't find them, substitute with whole white
   button mushrooms, with the stems removed)
2-3 cups of all-purpose flour
1 cup of nondairy milk + 1 tablespoon of apple cider vinegar
2 tablespoons of old bay seasoning
2 tablespoons of olive oil
Juice of 1 lemon (or 1 tablespoon of store-bought lemon juice)
Vegetable oil, for frying (at least 2½ cups)
Tomato slices and lettuce, for garnish (optional, but highly recommended)

Ingredients for Cocktail Sauce:

4 tablespoons of store-bought cocktail sauce
1 cup of **Basic Cashew Cream** (See Page 42)
1 teaspoon of salt
1 teaspoon of pepper
½ teaspoon of cayenne pepper

Directions

For Cocktail Sauce

1. In a medium-sized bowl, whisk all of the ingredients together until they turn into a
    uniform, creamy sauce.

2. Set aside.

Tip: Any extra sauce can be saved for additional recipes.

For Po' Boy

1. Drain the liquid from the cans of palm hearts (if using). Slice the stalks into large,
    token-sized pieces.

2. In a medium-sized bowl, whisk 1 tablespoon of the old bay, the lemon juice, and
    the olive oil together. Place the palm/mushrooms in the marinade and set aside
    to soak up the mixture.

3. In a deep pot or a fryer, add cooking oil to about 4 inches high (you should have enough to completely cover the top of the palms). While the oil is getting to temperature (between 385 to 400°F), set up your breading station.

4. Set up three bowls with the following:

   -Fill the first bowl with 1 cup of flour.
   -Add the cup of milk and vinegar mixture to the middle bowl.
   -In the last bowl, add 1 cup of flour mixed with the remaining tablespoon of old bay

5. Once oil reaches temperature and it is bubbling (but not smoking), it is ready for frying. Remove a palm/mushroom from the marinade and coat into the 1st bowl of flour. Next, dip into the liquid bowl, and finally, dip it in the bowl of seasoned flour. Place it in the fryer. Repeat this process with remaining pieces, being careful not to overcrowd the pot.

6. Using tongs or a metal, slotted spoon, fry the palms/mushrooms until they are golden on each side and crispy. Place them on a plate lined with a paper towel.

7. To assemble the po' boys, cut the baguettes in half and then slice lengthwise (like a bun).

   Tip: Toast the buns open-faced in a skillet with 1 tablespoon of vegan butter.

8. Spread the sauce on both the top and bottom of the baguette. Lay the hearts along the bottom half of the baguette. Then, add the lettuce and tomato to the top half (if using). Sprinkle extra salt and pepper to taste over the top (about ½ teaspoon each).

Desserts

Whoa, Oh Sweet Thang!

I usually stay away from desserts because, as Momma says, "I'm sweet enough"! All joking aside, even though I didn't inherit my mom's penchant for all things chocolate, I've been known to indulge in a brownie or two. Here are some of my favorite desserts, with just enough sweetness that Chaka Khan might have to do a remix:

- *Sea Salt Double-Dipped Chocolate Banana Butter Bites*
- *Chili Fruit Fondue Skewers*
- *Gluten-Free Sweet Potato Pie*
- *Red Velvet Cake Shake*
- *Apple Pie & Coconut Yogurt Parfait*
- *Fried Strawberry & Chocolate Sandwich Cookie Zepolis*
- *Banilly Vanilly, a Two-Ingredient Ice Cream!*
- *Mexican Hot Chocolate Brownies with Candied Orange Peel*
- *Banana Nut Hush Puppies*

Sea Salt Double-Dipped Chocolate Banana Butter Bites

Makes: 6 to 8 servings

Ingredients

2-3 bananas, slightly ripened
¼ to ½ cup of nut butter (such as peanut or almond butter)
1 medium-sized vegan dark chocolate bar (don't use baker's chocolate)
1½ cups of water
½ to 1 teaspoon of coarse sea salt (regular or fine sea salt works, too)
You will also need a utensil such as a skewer, toothpick, or turning fork!

Directions

1. Slice the bananas into 4 or 5 chunks per banana. Then slice each chunk in half so you have a top and bottom half. Keep each slice with its matching half.

2. Spread a small amount of nut butter (about ½ a teaspoon) on one slice of banana. Put its matching piece on top, like a sandwich.

3. Repeat this with the remaining bananas.

4. Add water to a medium saucepan over medium heat and bring to a boil.

5. Break the chocolate bar into 4 or 5 pieces. Make a double boiler to melt the chocolate by placing a medium-sized metal bowl or another saucepan on top of the pot of boiling water.

6. Using a rubber spatula, stir the chocolate bar gently in the bowl/pan to melt.

7. Once **half** of the chocolate has melted, turn off the heat and remove the bowl/pan from on top of the pot of boiling water. Continue to stir, making sure to scrape the sides. The residual heat will melt the rest of the chocolate.

8. Line a flat Tupperware-style container with parchment paper. Use a toothpick, skewer, or turning fork to dip each banana sandwich one at a time into the bowl of chocolate. Make sure to fully coat them. Place back in the container.

9. Repeat this with all the sandwiches. Garnish the chocolate-coated bites with the salt and freeze.

10. Wait at least 3 hours before enjoying. When ready, the banana turns into a nice, creamy ice cream texture.

Chili Fruit Fondue Skewers

Makes: 3 servings

Ingredients

6 skewers dipped in cold water (soak for 10 minutes)
6-10 fresh, whole strawberries
2 cups of fresh pineapple chunks (you can substitute with another "sturdy" type of fresh fruit)
1 teaspoon of smoked paprika
½ teaspoon of cayenne pepper
1 cup of Easy Chocolate Sauce (1 medium-sized vegan chocolate bar and 2 cups of water, for boiling)

Directions

1. Preheat your oven's broiler.

2. Lay the fruit flat on a cutting board (keep the strawberries whole). Sprinkle the spices onto all the fruit pieces.

3. Dip the skewers in cold water. Soak them for 10 minutes, then drain them on a napkin. Thread the skewers with the fruit alternating between the strawberries and pineapples on the same skewer.

4. Lay the spiced skewers on a baking sheet and place it in the broiler. You only want the fruit to slightly char but not to fully blacken (about 2-5 minutes, but closer to 3 or so).

5. **Make the chocolate sauce:** Add the water to a medium saucepan over medium heat and bring to a boil. Break the chocolate bar into 4 or 5 pieces. Make a double boiler to melt the chocolate by placing a medium-sized metal bowl or another saucepan on top of the pot of boiling water.

6. Using a rubber spatula, stir the chocolate bar gently in the bowl/pan to melt.

7. Once **half** of the chocolate has melted, turn the heat off, and remove the bowl/pan from the top of the pot of boiling water. Continue to stir, making sure to scrape the sides. The residual heat will melt the rest of the chocolate.

8. Pick 1 skewer and dip it in the chocolate to fully coat the fruit. Lay on a plate lined with parchment paper. Enjoy immediately, or try freezing for a chilly treat.

Gluten-Free Sweet Potato Pie

Makes: 6 to 8 servings

Ingredients

Ingredients for Crust:

1½ cups of gluten-free oats
½ of a ripe banana, smashed into almost a puree consistency
1 date, pitted and chopped
2 tablespoons of vegan butter
2 tablespoons raw sugar or other vegan sugar

Ingredients for Filling:

2-4 medium-sized sweet potatoes
½ cup almond milk
2 tablespoons of sugar
1 tablespoon of arrowroot
1 teaspoon of cinnamon
½ teaspoon of nutmeg

Ingredients for Candied Almond Topping:

¼ cup of sliced, raw almonds
1 teaspoon of lemon juice
½ teaspoon of cayenne
½ cup of simple syrup (equal parts sugar to water)

Directions

1. Boil the potatoes in salted water until soft and tender. You can leave the skin on until it's boiled. It comes off easier this way, so no need to peel! While potatoes are boiling, you can work on the crust.

2. Preheat oven to 375°F. In a dry blender, add all of the crust ingredients **EXCEPT** the vegan butter and banana. Pulse on a low-speed until the oats are just broken up (don't over blend or you'll get a meal). Add the banana and butter and blend until the mixture is slightly wet. Spoon the mixture into a well-oiled/sprayed pie pan and press down until you have an evenly distributed thin crust in the pan.

3. Bake the crust until it's no longer wet and the edges start to brown (about 12-15 minutes). Press down with your finger if you're not sure if it is done (it should be

slightly firm and no longer moist). Put crust to cool in your freezer while you work on your filling.

4. Remove the skins from your cooked potatoes. Smash the potatoes with a potato masher or heavy spoon. Add all of the filling ingredients **EXCEPT** the milk into the bowl with the potatoes and mix. Pour the milk and then the potato mixture into a blender. Blend until it is smooth, but with a consistency of a thick puree.

5. Pour the filling into the chilled crust and bake for about 40 minutes. You want the pie to be moist and thick, but not runny. Add a few more minutes if the pie isn't solid enough.

6. Season the almond slivers with the spice and lemon juice in a bowl. In a large skillet, heat the simple syrup on medium-low heat. Add the almonds and stir until they get candied and the syrup has evaporated. During the last 5 minutes of baking, top the pie with the candied almonds and put the pie back in the oven to brown them.

7. Let the pie cool for about 5 to 10 minutes and dig into that sucker!

Red Velvet Cake Shake

Makes: 2 servings

Ingredients

1 cup of frozen or fresh strawberries (if you use fresh, add a cup or so of ice)
1 banana
1 cup of nondairy milk (if you want to save calories, substitute with filtered water)
¼ cup cocoa powder*
1 tablespoon of agave (you can substitute with your preferred sweeter, such as maple syrup, 1 date, or raw sugar)
1 scoop of chocolate or vanilla protein powder (optional, but I like to feel healthier about my dessert by adding this)

*If you are not adding the protein powder, you may need to adjust the taste with your preferred sweetener

Directions

1. Pour the liquid into the blender.

2. Add the powders (if using) first, then all of the remaining ingredients.

3. Start with a low speed on your blender until it starts to "catch" and break down the ingredients.

4. Increase the speed to medium-high speed and blend until it takes on a thick milkshake consistency (about 1 minute or so).

5. Toast your health and enjoy!

Apple Pie & Coconut Yogurt Parfait

Makes : 2 to 4 servings*

*Servings will depend on how much yogurt you choose to use.

Ingredients

2 fresh apples, diced into small bites
1 tablespoon of vegan butter or margarine
¼ teaspoon of nutmeg (or use fresh whole nutmeg and just grate one whole one)
½ teaspoon of cinnamon
1 teaspoon of agave syrup or sugar
1 teaspoon of vanilla extract
1 cup of vegan granola
 Coconut or your favorite nondairy yogurt (this depends on how many parfaits you
 make, but use about ¾ to 1 cup for each parfait)

Directions

1. Heat the vegan butter in a large skillet over medium heat until it begins to melt. Add the apples and all of the other ingredients **EXCEPT** the yogurt and granola.

2. Mix well with a large spoon and brown for about 5-7 minutes, or until the mixture is soft and resembles apple pie filling.

3. To assemble the parfaits, place a large spoon full of granola on the bottom of a wine glass or a Mason jar. Next, add one spoonful of yogurt ensuring that you fully cover the granola. Follow the yogurt with a layer of the apple filling.

4. Continue this process until you have several layers and the glass is full.

5. Top with a little more filling.

Fried Strawberry & Chocolate Sandwich Cookie Zepolis

Makes: 6 to 8 servings

Ingredients

1 pack of vegan pizza dough (set at room temperature for 30 minutes)
10-15 vegan chocolate Oreo-style sandwich cookies
A handful of fresh, sliced strawberries
½ to 1 cup of all-purpose flour
Oil, for frying (at least 2 cups)
1-2 tablespoons of powdered sugar

Directions

1. Remove the store-bought dough from the fridge. Let it set on a counter at room temperature for 30 minutes.

2. Twist open the sandwich cookies and place a strawberry slice in between each one.

3. In a large pot or fryer, heat 2-3 cups of vegetable oil. When it reaches 375 to 400°F, it is ready for frying. While the oil is reaching temp, prep the zepolis.

4. Lightly flour a surface. Flour a rolling pin (or a wine bottle works if you don't have a rolling pin) and roll out the dough to stretch. Tear off a piece of the dough big enough to wrap around a cookie completely. Drape the dough around a cookie. Repeat this step with the remaining cookies.

5. When the oil has reached temp, drop the dough wrapped cookies in the oil. Be careful not to overcrowd the pan.

6. Use tongs or a metal slotted spoon to turn over the zepolis. Let them get golden brown on each side. They should also puff up and bubble after about 3-5 minutes.

7. Remove them from the heat and drain them on a napkin-lined plate. Top with the powdered sugar and serve immediately.

Banilly Vanilly, a Two-Ingredient Ice Cream!

Makes: 4 servings

Ingredients

4 frozen bananas, sliced
2 teaspoons of vanilla extract

Tip: If it is not blending well, add small amounts of water or nondairy milk at a time, and as needed. Do not overuse the liquid, or you will not get the ice cream consistency.

Directions

1. If you haven't already, chop the bananas into coin-sized pieces or chunks and freeze them in a container for at least 3 hours.

2. Remove the bananas from the freezer, place them in a blender and add the vanilla.

3. Blend together, starting at a low speed to initially break down the bananas into smaller bits. Then, gradually increase the speed (but not to the highest speed). If your blender is having trouble, add a little bit of the liquid.

4. Serve with fruit, with crushed cookies, or in a cone.

5. Stores in the freezer at least a month.

Mexican Hot Chocolate Brownies with Candied Orange Peel

In Texas, when you hear the words "Mexican hot chocolate" you just know you are gonna get that spicy, chocolatey, cinnamon or nutmeg kind of flavor. This is my signature dessert, and you can be sure it's a hit!

Makes: 6 to 10 servings

Ingredients

2 ¼ cups of flour
1 cup of water
¾ cup of cocoa powder
½ cup of vegan butter or margarine, melted
1 cup of sugar
1 teaspoon of salt
½ teaspoon of baking powder
1 teaspoon of cayenne pepper
1 teaspoon of cinnamon

Ingredients for Candied Orange Peel:

1 orange peel, cut into thin strips
¼ cup of water
2 teaspoons of raw sugar or other sugar

Directions

1. Preheat the oven to 350°F.

2. Pour 1 cup of flour with 1 cup of water into a medium saucepan over low heat. Stir constantly with a fork or rubber spatula until you have a gluey consistency.

3. In a small, separate pan, melt the vegan butter. Once melted, add it to a large bowl with the sugar, salt, and cocoa powder. Mix thoroughly. Add the gluey flour mixture to this bowl and mix well. Add the remaining (dry flour), cayenne, cinnamon, and baking powder to the bowl and mix thoroughly with a large spoon or rubber spatula until you have a nice batter.

4. Spread the batter in a square greased pan and bake for 25-30 minutes. Place a toothpick or a tip of a knife down the middle to check the doneness. Let the brownies cool while you make the candied orange peel.

For Candied Orange Peel

1. Wash off an orange, and peel off the rind. Slice into very thin long strips.

2. In a medium saucepan, whisk ¼ cup of water with 1 teaspoon of sugar and bring to a boil. Once the simple syrup has started to boil and get a bit sticky, add in the orange strips and coat with the syrup. Stir the peel constantly with a fork.

3. Once all the liquid has been absorbed and the pieces are a tender, candy-like consistency (about 3 minutes), add the last teaspoon of sugar to the pot and stir for an additional minute. Remove from the heat and top the brownies with the candy.

4. Any extra candy stores for a few days in a sandwich bag.

Banana Nut Hush Puppies

This Southern classic is often served for breakfast or dessert, and may even come as a side dish at some food joints in Texas; although, those puppies would be savory! This sweeter version, made with bananas, adds a nice moistness to this traditional treat.

Makes: 6 to 10 servings

Ingredients

1 cup of corn meal
½ cup of almond milk
½ cup of banana puree (1 banana blended until smooth)
1 teaspoon of sea salt
1 teaspoon of baking powder
1 teaspoon of sugar
1 **FLEGG** (1 tablespoon of ground flaxseed + 3 tablespoons of warm water)
½ cup of crushed nuts (I used cashews because that's what I had on hand)
1-2 cups of vegetable oil, for frying

Directions

1. Add all of the dry ingredients in a large bowl and whisk together. In a separate bowl, add all the wet ingredients **EXCEPT** the oil and whisk together. Add the wet into the dry and stir with a large spoon to create a thick batter.

2. Preheat the oil in a fryer or deep pot. Once the oil reaches around 380°F, your oil is ready for frying.

3. Using a medium-sized spoon, begin to drop little balls of batter into the hot oil. Brown them completely on each side. This should be about 3-5 minutes total, depending on how big you make the balls. If you aren't sure if they are fully cooked, then break one open to see if they are done. When done, the hush puppies should be golden brown on the outside and fluffy on the inside. They should not be moist or batter-like inside.

4. Drain the puppies on a napkin, cool, and serve!

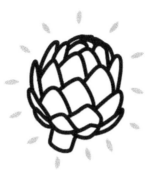

CHAPTER NINE

EATING OUT

Although I personally enjoy the control of cooking for yourself and really putting that love on a plate, you can still get some quality food that's vegan while dining out. You can also continue to socialize and eat out without having that anxiety of "I ain't never gone get them to eat at a vegan restaurant with me." While more and more restaurants expand on their plant based menu offerings, many cuisines around the world traditionally offer a wide variety of meals that are already free from animal ingredients. There are also sites to help you find vegan or vegan-friendly restaurants.

Sites such as www.happycow.net or simply doing a search on YELP! are good places to get intel on what your vegan options are out there and how good those options are.

For fast food options and much more the following are also good options for restaurant guides in your area:

veganuary.com/eating-out

veganeatingout.com

The following is a brief summary of types of restaurants and diverse cuisines from various parts of the world and what to look for in case you find yourself in a position where you were unable to pre-plan your outing:

Steakhouses: Clearly, not the most plant-based friendly, but you can usually get a decent salad – just order one without egg, croutons, and cheese.

Seafood: Next to a steakhouse, seafood restaurants are probably the least vegan-friendly. However, you can ask your server for an order of pasta with olive oil and grilled veggies.

Middle Eastern Food: The sides and pitas are typically vegan with the exception of things like tzatziki sauce, which are made with yogurt. Some restaurants offer falafel, which are made from chickpeas, and are usually vegan.

Mexican Food: There is definitely lots to choose from in Mexican restaurants starting with the chips and salsa! Most places also offer veggie fajitas with guacamole and corn or flour tortillas. You can also order veggie tacos without cheese. Black beans and rice or refried beans are also good options. Just confirm that lard and/or chicken stock are not used in the beans or rice. However, you should be safe if these items are also in the vegetarian section of the menu. At times, sour cream is added to the guacamole, so let your waiter know "no cheese or sour cream" on your orders.

Thai Food: Thai meals that are typically vegan-friendly include Pad-Thai and tofu dishes. Be sure to ask if their vegetarian items are made with fish sauce as a precaution. Also, request "no egg" in any of your meals.

Chinese Food: Chinese restaurants usually offer a vast selection of vegan meals. Stir-fry w/ tofu or bean curd, General Tso's Tofu, Mao Poo Tofu, and vegetable rice bowls are good options. If you see a vegetarian dish made with oyster sauce, simply request that they use soy sauce instead. Also, stick to boiled rice, as fried rice is usually made with egg.

Ethiopian Food: Traditionally, Ethiopian lentil and bean dishes are usually vegan. Just be sure to request "no butter" for your meals just in case.

Italian Restaurants: You definitely won't go hungry in an Italian restaurant! You can try pasta with marinara sauce or oil and garlic, as well as vegetable pizza without cheese (this may seem odd, but you'll soon find out who makes the best pizza crust veggie pizzas in town, as flavor is everything!). For pasta dishes, do ask your waiter if they make the pasta fresh in house with eggs. Otherwise, the pasta is usually vegan if they use dry pasta.

Breakfast Diners: Not the best choice for plant based eating, but there are always options, such as toast or bagels with jelly or margarine, fruit bowls, hash browns, grits, or oatmeal with nondairy milk.

Mediterranean Restaurants: Good options include hummus & pita bread, falafel, Greek salad without the feta, tabouli, and couscous.

Indian Restaurants: Indian cuisine offers delicious and flavorful vegan options. It can be a bit tricky at first as many of their creamy sauces contain dairy (or ghee). However, tomato based dishes work well. Vegetable samosas are great appetizers while a go-to dish is Channa Masala, which are curried chickpeas. Dosas and "Dhal" (lentil dishes) are also good options. You can order boiled rice or pilau rice, as well as nans and chapatis (types of breads to dip in our main dish) to complement your meal.

Bar Food: If you've ever spent time at a bar and drank to the point of starvation, you know all about "old faithful" a.k.a. French fries! As far as bar food, this could be your only option. If you are a conscious drinker and want something light instead, you could order a side salad with balsamic dressing.

Fast Foods & Chain Restaurants: Most of these types of venues, particularly in major cities, do have a vegan menu. Simply ask your waiter for the menu or check on their website for a list of their plant based offerings.

Other Tips

- Beware of vegetarian restaurants— particularly older ones— that may use dairy and eggs in their dishes, as vegetarian does not mean the same as vegan.
- Some casual dining restaurants may have icons at the bottom of their menus and next to specific menu items to signal vegan dishes. Often times, vegetarian dishes can also be veganized.
- If you live in an area that doesn't have a vegan restaurant or vegan options, politely encourage local restaurants to include a few options via email or by filling-out a comment. This will be helpful to do, as restaurants are always towards becoming more versatile and to increase their clientele.
- Above all, don't be scared to ask questions! Your ethics and health are too important not to.

CHAPTER TEN

LIFE EVENTS

We work hard and sometimes we want to play hard too. We always got something going on. Whether it's a baby shower, wedding, company party, cook-outs, or block parties, eating a plant-based diet will not prevent you from enjoying your life.

Here are some things that you can eat at some of those events:

- guacamole or salsa and corn chips
- hummus plates with pita or vegetables
- fruit plates
- nuts
- grilled vegetable kabobs
- butterless popcorn (FYI, most movie theater popcorn doesn't have butter on it until they pump it on. Many theaters actually use vegan margarine instead of butter, so check your local theater. You may be able to enjoy your popcorn – butter and all!)
- and many more!

You can also eat before you go, and just enjoy the drinks (Hello!).

Most importantly, **bring your own.** Show off those new cooking skills you've learned! Bringing your own means you'll definitely have options.

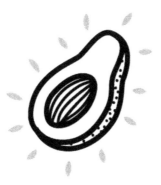

CHAPTER ELEVEN

OTHER RESOURCES

Choosing to begin a new lifestyle journey is to embark on a new learning curve as well. How can you easily unlearn habits that took a lifetime to create? Although by this point, you will have the food part in check, it is often the *will* and *desire* that is the toughest part. This is why I would recommend continuing on your new path by doing your own research in terms of what veganism is and what it means with regards to an ethical lifestyle. Veganism is not just about food, since nonhuman animals are also exploited for things like body products, clothing, and entertainment. I feel that it is important to know where certain companies stand (or don't) in terms of their business practices and their treatment of nonhuman animals, as well as their workers. Don't let your journey stop here. Our individual choices do make a difference, and they add up when we make those choices collectively.

Here are a few suggestions for support and general resources to help you continue on your journey:

✓ **Vegan Registered Dieticians and Resource Groups**

The Vegan RD: theveganrd.com
Vegetarian Resource Group: vrg.org
Facebook Group: *Ask a Vegan Dietician**

*Registered dieticians help answer questions related to diet free of charge.

✓ **Documentaries**

Earthlings
Forks Over Knives
Vegucated
Cowspiracy
Unity
Speciesism: The Movie
Peaceable Kingdom

✓ **General Websites**

My Own Recipe & Blog: thevvc.com
Veganism of Color: veganismofcolor.org
Food Empowerment Project: foodispower.org
Sistah Vegan Project: sistahvegan.com

✓ **General Web Groups**

It is also important to know that someone else out there understands where you are coming from and can completely empathize with you. I am extremely blessed to have a partner and friends that are either vegan themselves, or are vegan allies and are more than happy to eat plant-based foods when they are with me. I do understand that this may not be the case for you, so you may find the following groups helpful for support and may even find some vegan homies out there near you:

vegweb.com

veggieboards.com

Search your local Facebook for a group near you. You may also be interested in the following groups and pages for basic questions or support:

- Vegan Beginners 101
- Afro Vegan Society
- Vegan Hip Hop Movement
- What Phat Vegans Eat

✓ **Online Shops**

Vegan Essentials: veganessentials.com is one of my favorites, but there are many more vegan online shops depending on your region and country of residence.

✓ **Support Your Local Farms and Markets**

blackfarmers.org
coopdirectory.org
localharvest.org/csa
sustainabletable.org

✓ **Books to Read**

- *Vegan Soul Kitchen* by Bryant Terry

- *Never Too Late to Go Vegan*
  by Carol J. Adams, Patti Breitman, and Virginia Messina

- *By Any Greens Necessary* by Tracey Lynn McQuirter, MPH

- *The Complete Guide to Vegan Food Substitutions*
  by Celine Steen & Joni Marie Newman

- *Sistah Vegan* by Dr. A. Breeze Harper

- *Veganism in an Oppressive World*
  by Julia Feliz Brueck, A Vegans-of-Color Community Project

- *Baby and Toddler Vegan Feeding Guide*
  by Julia Feliz Brueck (dietician approved, evidence based, and helpful for those with kids!)

- *Uncommon Fruits & Vegetables*
  by Elizabeth Schneider (this book will help you with using many types of exotic produce you may not be familiar with; it truly inspires me)

- *Homemade Vegan Pantry* by Miyoko Schinner

✓ **Magazines**

T.O.F.U. Magazine
Laika Magazine
Vegan Lifestyle Mag
Thrive Magazine

...and many more!

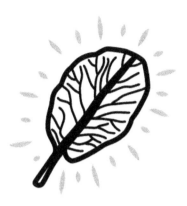

CHAPTER TWELVE

MOVE YA ASS!

Initially, when I went vegetarian (and later vegan), I started to care more about my overall well-being and started to do physical activities for my health as well. I actually found myself enjoying them too (although, I still hate to run!) and open to trying new types of exercises and sports. Fifteen years after graduating from high school (please don't do the math!), I have more energy and vitality than I did back then. I accredit this to realizing that health is about much more than just diet, clothes size, or appearance. For me, it is about being mindful of what you put in it and how you treat it as you go along in life. I decided to add this section should any of my readers need a little inspiration in this department as a complement to embracing an ethical lifestyle change and plant-based eating.

So, if you are able, now that you got your eating down, then it's time to "move ya ass"! Just a note before we start though...

Always check with your doctor on the types of physical activities that you can take part in, especially if you have health conditions that may be aggravated by physical exertion.

The following are routines that have worked for me, an abled bodied person. I recognize that not everyone will be able to just get up and work out, and I encourage folks with disabilities and health conditions to find what works for them— if their disability and wellbeing allows.

Getting Started

You may think that going from zero to 100 is a bit unrealistic, but you aren't starting at zero! Even steps during your typical daily routine are steps in the right direction, so if you are walking, you already started. For me, the first step to getting more active was by keeping track of a pedometer (a step tracker), writing down my steps accomplishments daily, and challenging myself week after week to do better than I had done the week before. I even had a chart on my office door as a physical reminder, which helped to keep me accountable to myself.

Most phones have a built-in app that works as a pedometer, so you most likely already have one. Otherwise, you can find simple ones at dollar type stores for a few dollars, and larger chain stores (you know the ones!) will also carry different kinds that you can clip on yourself.

Either way, you don't even need a pedometer, as long as you just make a commitment to yourself to get more active *for you*.

Here a few simple things you can do to get in a few extra steps in throughout the day:

- Park farther away when on a quick outing or when going to work.
- Take the stairs instead of the elevator.
- Actively play at the park with your kids or friends. You can incorporate some cheap outdoor toys like foam guns, Velcro mittens, and frisbees to get you moving.
- Instead of email alerts, walk to deliver the letters or memos at the office.
- If you are tracking your steps, challenge friends to get on board and make a game out of it.
- Walk around in the mall; it's air-conditioned!
- Discover the nature in your area. Take a walk through the wilderness and learn about your local wildlife.
- If you have a show you enjoy watching, you can get some steps in or even some jumping jacks during commercial breaks.
- Think about other types of activities you enjoy and how to incorporate extra movement in them.

More Intense Workouts

If you'd like to try a more involved exercise routine, you can do so from the comfort of your own home. Forget the bourgeoisie workout clothes, and get fit in ya draws, y'all!

If you have a smartphone, you already know that there are thousands of apps on them to make life easier. One of my favorite apps, which makes my exercise routine much more convenient, is "My Fitness Pal'. It's like having a gym (with a trainer) in your pocket. You can customize workouts, put in the amount of time you have, the level of difficulty, and whatever else you need. With this information, it will generate a workout just for you. Pretty dope, right? The damn thing will even talk to you and coach you through the whole routine! The best thing about it is that most of the workouts are accessible without needing any gym equipment (such as dumbbells, for example) since you work with your own bodyweight and calisthenics (exercise based on body movements).

If you don't have access to a phone, you can search for exercise routines on YouTube university, as I like to call it.

If it is accessible to you, perhaps finding a gym would be most helpful? Many gyms offer free weekly passes so that you can get a taste of what their facilities have to offer. During that free trial, trainers will give you a tour and even free sessions to get you comfortable and to teach you how to properly use their equipment and facilities. You can get these free passes on the websites of various gyms, as well as in wellness and vitamin shops, usually by their cash registers. Some stores even have community boards where local trainers advertise their services; you may find some low-cost exercise groups in them, as well.

Other Sources of Free or Damn Near-Free Fitness Classes

- Library (look out for community events and local bulletin announcements)
- Local Parks & Rec
- Keep an eye on Facebook Events
- Yelp! (this has become my counsel, counselor, judge, and more - YELP's word is bond!)
- Groupon (find cheap deals on creative workout activities that you can go half on with friends or family)
- Running stores (they usually have free events or running groups advertised)
- Community pool
- Athletic stores (ask about "Brand Ambassadors;" they organize free or cheap classes in the community)

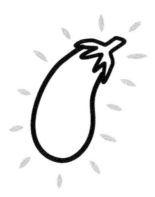

CHAPTER THIRTEEN

THAT'S A WRAP!

My love for my family and the Southern traditions that centered around our meals while growing up and my desire for better health are the fuel that allowed me to create this book.

I hope that you will share all that you have learned within these pages to create your own fond memories around plant-based eating, and perhaps continue to ponder how your daily choices affect others, yourself, and our future on this planet.

May this book make your journey a little easier and fill it with lots of *soul!*

ABOUT THE AUTHOR

Cametria Hill is a culinary professional specialized as a personal chef, caterer, and food blogger. Before her recent move to Los Angeles, the last 14 years in Brooklyn saw Cametria perfecting her cooking skills in some of the most renowned NYC vegan companies and food festivals, which included The Seed Market, Yeah Dawg!, and the greatly popular food truck, The Cinnamon Snail.

Growing up in Houston, Texas afforded Cametria the opportunity to surround herself by what she has designated as the four best food types on Earth: Mexican, Soul Food, BBQ, and Cajun. Influenced by these culinary treasures, Cametria masterfully transformed and merged them into her own deliciously crafted plant-based Southern innovations.

Also a freelance journalist, content creator, and multi-media artist, when she's not producing or in the kitchen, Cametria can be found immersed on the guitar or enjoying documentaries which she is admittedly obsessed with.

Get to know Cametria and connect with her via:

Blog: thevvc.com

Facebook: SouthernGirlsGuideToPlantBasedEating & CamThaVeg

Instagram: CamThaVeg

Tumblr: CamThaVeg

Twitter: CamThaVeg

CPSIA information can be obtained
at www.ICGtesting.com
Printed in the USA
LVHW061622030119
602636LV00010B/330/P

9 780998 994628